Ear Acupuncture

Understanding the illustrations

The 'open' ear: Used to show the location of the various ear acupuncture points. Those points that are hidden when looking straight at the ear are sometimes shown in an 'open' ear. In such illustrations the edges of the helix, tragus and antitragus are folded back and held in place with hooks so that the subtragus, the inside of the antitragus and the inside of the edge of the helix become visible. In reality, no hooks would be used, of course.

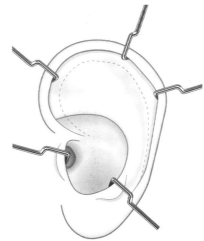

Different symbols are used to indicate the points:

- A bullet point means that the point is visible when viewed straight on.
- A triangle means that the point is concealed, i.e. lies on the inside of – for example – the tragus, or behind the edge of the helix.
- A star means that the point lies on the wall between the antihelix and the concha.

The placing of the points in the illustrations is schematic. Because no two ears are the same it is difficult to give an exact location. To actually locate active points in each individual ear, careful point finding is recommended.

Commissioning Editor: *Karen Morley*
Development Editor: *Kerry McGechie*
Project Manager: *Susan Stuart*
Designer: *Stewart Larking*
Illustration Manager: *Merlyn Harvey*
Illustrator: *Graeme Chambers*

Ear Acupuncture

Kajsa Landgren

Acupuncturist, Helsingborg, Sweden

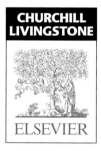

CHURCHILL
LIVINGSTONE

ELSEVIER

Edinburgh   London   New York   Oxford   Philadelphia   St Louis   Sydney   Toronto 2008

CHURCHILL LIVINGSTONE

An imprint of Elsevier Limited

First and second edition published in Swedish under the title Öronakupunktur
1. First edition 2004
2. Second edition 2006
© Kajsa Landgren

First edition published in English
© 2008, Elsevier Limited. All rights reserved.

First edition 2004
Second edition 2006
English First edition 2008

ISBN: 9780443068997

British Library Cataloguing in Publication Data
A catalogue record for this book is available from the British Library

Library of Congress Cataloging in Publication Data
A catalog record for this book is available from the Library of Congress

Notice
Neither the Publisher nor the Author assume any responsibility for any loss or injury and/or damage to persons or property arising out of or related to any use of the material contained in this book. It is the responsibility of the treating practitioner, relying on independent expertise and knowledge of the patient, to determine the best treatment and method of application for the patient.

The Publisher

ELSEVIER your source for books, journals and multimedia in the health sciences
www.elsevierhealth.com

Working together to grow libraries in developing countries

www.elsevier.com | www.bookaid.org | www.sabre.org

ELSEVIER   BOOK AID International   Sabre Foundation

The Publisher's policy is to use **paper manufactured from sustainable forests**

Printed in China

Contents

Contents

Contents

Preface

I have studied and practised ear acupuncture for 19 years and for the past 12 have taught the method, which I find ever more fascinating.

This book is concerned just with the basics of ear acupuncture: how to diagnose illness by examining the ear, how to find the active points, and how to carry out treatment in accord with the principles of auricular therapy. You can get good results with ear acupuncture without having to buy advanced and costly technical equipment and without having to study traditional Chinese medicine. Ear acupuncture is a simple reflex theory based on the idea that each part of the body and each organ has a corresponding point in the ear, which, in the event of malfunction, can be treated to relieve pain and restore health. Knowledge of the ear's reflex zones, adequate time for examination and common sense are all that are needed to achieve impressive results.

I have benefited from hearing various teachers describe what ear acupuncture is all about. At a very early stage in my studies I realised that there was no consensus on exactly where each ear acupuncture point is located, the function it has and the name it should be given. As I studied Chinese and Western books and texts, ancient and modern, there was initial uncertainty but with time my understanding grew and eventually I found I could tell the wood from the trees.

This book is based on the knowledge I have thus far accumulated. My goal has been to follow major themes and make logical connections, to reconcile seemingly contradictory observations with what I have found to work well in my clinic and to summarise when there is general agreement among experts. Points which other authors may consider to be two separate entities, located a millimetre or so from one another I have represented as one point, or zone. It's possible that on occasion I have gone too far in my eagerness to simplify. However, the acupuncturist should stick to the basic principle of treating active points. The fact that they are active, surely, is of greater importance than the name they bear.

This book is a teaching manual and can be used as a reference work in the acupuncturist's daily work. But some sections are of a more general nature and may be read by people with only a passing interest in ear acupuncture.

It is aimed at several different groups of readers: at body acupuncturists who wish to find out more about ear acupuncture; at doctors, nurses, midwives and physiotherapists who wish to learn an additional method of treatment; at reflexologists who may wish to compare ear acupuncture with their own methods; and at patients who would like a greater understanding of the treatment they have chosen or are considering choosing.

My ambition has been to write in plain, easy to understand language so the book may be understood by readers with no prior medical knowledge. Certain basic phenomena are described more than once in different sections of the book. The idea is that the book need not be read in order, from cover to cover but can be used both as a manual and for reference.

We live in a dynamic, ever-changing world. Colossal amounts of information are available via books, articles, databases and on the internet. Knowledge of acupuncture, like other medical science, is in a state of continual change and development. Moreover, ear acupuncture is a new science in comparison with body acupuncture; much remains to be discovered. New findings are bound to be published that can add to your knowledge. So keep your eyes — and ears! — open.

I would like to thank all those who have made this book possible. My parents for their belief in me and encouragement in all I do. My husband Dennis and our children Arvid, Axel and Ellen for their patience in putting up with my writing — their presence gave me the peace and stimulation needed to bring the book to fruition. Maya was a great help with the chapters I wrote in Tuscany and a great many other people, among them Linda Kvist, have inspired and encouraged me.

A special thanks to Chris Mosey for translating the original text into English.

Kajsa Landgren

The history of ear acupuncture

The basic theory of ear acupuncture is that certain points in the ear have an effect on other organs, body parts or functions. Ear acupuncture is a treatment involving stimulation of these points to prevent and treat illness and relieve pain.

In France, where modern ear acupuncture was refined and developed in the 1950s, the method became known as *auriculothérapie* — in English 'auricular therapy' — a term which combines the Latin words for 'ear' and 'treatment'. In this book I shall use the simpler expression 'ear acupuncture'.

Ear acupuncture is a concept that embraces both diagnosis — examination of the ear to find 'active points', and treatment — the stimulation of these active points with acupuncture needles, semi-permanent needles[1] or with pellets.[2]

Ear acupuncture is a variation of body acupuncture and forms a small, independent part of the greater science. The principles of ear acupuncture treatment are different from those of body acupuncture. Ear acupuncture can be used in combination with body acupuncture, or as a separate treatment.

Acupuncture literally means 'to prick with needles'. The method has been used for thousands of years in Asia. Along with pulse and tongue diagnosis (see Ch. 2, A brief look at traditional Chinese medicine), characteristic of Chinese medicine, Chinese doctors also treated conditions such as high temperature and pain by massaging the ear, by burning points in it or by controlled bleeding using needles. To this day, such methods remain part of Chinese folk medicine.

The basic idea of modern ear acupuncture is that every part of the body has a corresponding reflex point in the ear, which can be used both for diagnosis and treatment. If something is out of balance in the body,

---

[1] A small needle that can remain in place for several days.
[2] Metal 'press pellets' or sometimes organic seeds held in place with band aid.

this will be reflected in the particular part of the ear. The reflex point can be sore or change colour. If exactly that point in the ear is treated, the corresponding part of the body reacts in a positive fashion. The ear's active points may be linked to form the figure of a tiny human being turned upside down. This theory was launched by the French doctor Paul Nogier in the 1950s. What he described was a so-called reflex zone system.

Ear acupuncture in ancient China

The roots of traditional Chinese medicine (TCM) go back at least 4000 years (see Ch. 2, A brief look at traditional Chinese medicine). Part of the basic thinking behind acupuncture is described in texts that are more than 2000 years old. To a large degree, these deal with treatment using herbs and body acupuncture, but they also mention the importance of the ear in diagnosis and treatment of illness. TCM developed in a multicultural society plagued with war and divisions and with no uniform system of medicine.

In ancient China points in the ear were used in no apparent order. The Chinese did not discover that the reflex points were divided up according to a special system, reflecting the organs and body parts they represent.

The ear as an aid to diagnosis

The *Nei Jing*, or *Huang Di Nei Jing Su Wen*, medical classic of the Yellow Emperor; the Yellow Emperor's Canon of Medicine, was written by several authors around 403-221 BC, a period of great internal strife in China. It gives detailed descriptions of points, meridians, indications and counterindications and describes different types of needles and manipulation techniques. It provides a unique record of the basic theory of traditional Chinese medicine and of the collected medical knowledge of the era. The book takes the form of conversations between the emperor and the court physician. The emperor poses questions on health, illness and treatment; the physician replies. Included in the *Nei Jing*, among other things, is the assertion that the ear may be inspected to make diagnoses concerning the kidney.[3] The book also describes how each of the six yang meridians[4] has a connection to the ear. Yang meridians connect in pairs to yin meridians. Therefore even yin organs have contact with the ear. According to Chinese thinking, all meridians are united in this fashion in the ear.

In the book *The Story of Chinese Acupuncture and Moxibustion* (Fu 1975) we read: 'The Canon of Medicine (Nei Jing) describes the intricate links between the pinna and the other organs and notes that any physiological or pathological change in the heart, kidney, brain, liver, spleen or small and large intestines may be reflected on the pinna'.

During the Sung dynasty (960–1279 AD) diagnoses were made by inspecting and palpating the ear. In the 13th century (under the Yuan dynasty), the book *Wei*

---

[3] In TCM the kidney was seen as 'opening' in the ear, meaning that hereditary weakness (in either the kidney itself or in the energy field around it) can be reflected in the actual shape of the ear, for example in the case of a small, thin earlobe, or ears that are smaller or placed lower than average. All symptoms of illness in the ear — for example impaired hearing and tinnitus — can, according to the same theory, be linked to a weakness in the kidney. See Ch. 2, A brief look at traditional Chinese medicine (TCM).

[4] In TCM everything is divided into the two polarities of yin and yang. All organs and energy channels, or meridians, are either yin or yang.

Sheng Pao Chien described in greater detail how yin and yang, the five elements and the inner organs were related to the ear.

Wexu (1985) quotes the *Zen Zhi Zhun Sheng* (Book of Symptoms and Their Treatment): 'A bright and shiny coloration of the helix[5] of the ear is a sign of good vitality. On the contrary, if the helix is extremely dry, death is not far off… If the ear is thin and pale, the homolateral kidney is ill'.

From diagnosis to treatment

Body acupuncture traces its ancestry further back in time than ear acupuncture. Before man began mining metal, acupuncture points were worked with needles of stone, bone, ceramic fragments or bamboo chips. Later needles were made of bronze and steel. From 200 AD, needles were also made of gold and silver.

Knowledge of how illness may be diagnosed with the aid of the external ear is preserved in records dating back more than 2000 years. Several centuries later various authors described methods of treating the ear.

In the book *Prescriptions for Emergencies*, written in 300 AD, Ko Hung describes how one might blow in a patient's ears as a way of treating suffocation.[6] The book also presents an older doctor's considered opinion that the juice of a leek should be poured into the ear in the event of 'sudden death with eyes closed'. In 600 AD, during the Tang dynasty, jaundice and other epidemics were treated with acupuncture and the burning of moxa in the external ear. A book from 700 AD[7] contains the recommendation to fill the patient's ear with 'bolted snake skin' in the event of malaria. Children suffering from cramp were treated by burning moxa on the back of the ear.

Moxa and bleeding techniques

In 1572, during the Ming dynasty (1368–1644 AD), a book was published on the eight extra meridians (*The study of eight special meridians*), in which the relationship between the meridians and the ear was further developed. During the same period the *Great compendium of acupuncture and moxibustion* was written. This is concerned not just with body acupuncture but also provides more information on ear acupuncture. It tells how the apex, or top, of the ear can be burnt with moxa[8] or bled in the treatment of hepatitis and bloodshot eyes.

This sort of knowledge has existed for centuries in Chinese folk medicine. Bloodshot eyes are still treated by an acupuncturist using a needle to cause a little bleeding in the ear. It is also common for the ear to be massaged, for example in the event of headaches.

Several other ancient Chinese texts, in addition those named here, describe a connection between energy channels and the ear and claim that different illnesses may be treated by sticking a needle in the ear, making a point in the ear bleed or by creating a little burn sore at the point. Although ear acupuncture was used in China, the method did not develop into any separate technique or as a special form of therapy as

---

[5] The helix is the outermost part of the ear, the 'rolled' edge surrounding the ear.
[6] Taken from *Ear acupuncture. A Chinese medical report. The complete text of the Nanking army ear acupuncture team*, written in the 1960s and translated into English in 1974 (Huang 1974).
[7] *The Prescriptions of Treating Malaria*, by Chen Tsang-chi, born c. 730 AD.
[8] Moxa is a herb used to keep the patient warm. Bleeding allowed for several drops of blood to be extracted, by sticking a needle in one of the points of the ear. For more on moxa treatment see Ch. 2, A brief look at traditional Chinese medicine (TCM) and Ch. 11, Method.

it was to do in Europe. Ear acupuncture was an integrated part of traditional Chinese medicine, an aid to diagnosis and one of several methods of treatment.

Acupuncture out of favour in China

In 1822 the authorities in China issued a directive that acupuncture should no longer be practised. Modern Western medical methods, which had by now reached China, would replace traditional Chinese medicine, which was seen as being outmoded and unscientific. When the emperor's family ceased to use acupuncture, the Chinese universities in which it was taught were closed. And even after the last emperor abdicated in 1911, Western influence continued to grow. The knowledge of acupuncture was passed down among families with a medical tradition, however, and acupuncture lived on, along with herbal treatment, in folk medicine.

Acupuncture regains its position in China

In the newly created Republic of China Western medicine was seen as being more soundly based scientifically than TCM. Pöyhönen (1996) writes: 'As late as 1941 leading Marxists considered traditional medicine to be "rubbish collected over thousands of years" but just 17 years later Mao Zedong came up with a new and contradictory formulation: "Traditional Chinese medicine is a great treasure house which ought to be explored and further enriched."' When Mao took over China in 1949 the health of its people was in a bad way. One way of quickly bringing about an improvement was the re-establishment of TCM and for it to be used in tandem with Western medicine. Universities in TCM were reopened and there was investment in research and documentation of the effects of acupuncture. A large corps of so called 'barefoot doctors' was formed. These doctors didn't have a complete medical education but they could treat simpler forms of illness and give advice on hygiene and health. The barefoot doctors were sent out all over the country, so that people in the cities and the countryside would have access to health care. Ear acupuncture was popularised by the barefoot doctors, the more so because it was a form of acupuncture that was considerably easier and quicker to learn than body acupuncture. A description of the method for treating the apex of the ear in cases of hepatitis and eye problems is, for example, to be found in an instruction book written in 1968 for the barefoot doctors (Silverstein et al., 1975).

The development of ear acupuncture in China

The French doctor Paul Nogier is considered to be the father of modern ear acupuncture (his breakthrough is described later in this chapter). When Nogier's article on the ear's reflex points was published in China in 1958, his ideas won wide acceptance but in Chinese articles it was pointed out that research into ear acupuncture was already advanced in China at the time Nogier published his findings. In 1956, for example, the Health Department in Shangtung Province reported that ear acupuncture could cure 'throat numbness' and a major study of more than two thousand patients was made at the close of the 1950s by the Nanking army ear acupuncture research team. The team searched for active reflex points in patients' ears[9] and documented the effect of acupuncture on them.

---

[9] Active reflex points are points which become tender with palpation or have changed electrical resistance and which represent the organ or part of the body troubling the patient (see Ch. 7, Reflect points).

The Story of Chinese Acupuncture and Moxibustion (Fu 1975) describes ear acupuncture thus:

> *Modern development of the therapy began in 1956 when the Laihsi County Hospital in Shantung Province obtained marked results in treating acute tonsillitis by the old folk practice of pinna needling. In 1957 … doctors effectively treated stye and some other eye diseases by pricking on the back of the pinna, causing slight bleeding. Research and clinical practice by Chinese medical units resulted after 1958 in a greater versatility in pinna needling. It was found effective not only in alleviating headache, toothache, backache, neuralgia, colic pain of gall bladder and kidneys, and relieving pain during skin incision, but also to treat insomnia, hypertension, ulcers and enuresis, among other diseases. Probing or direct inspection of the pinna was also found to be an aid in diagnosis.*

The Nanking army ear acupuncture research team wrote in 1972 (Huang 1974):

> *In the last few years we went through several hundred thousand treatments, cured more than 200 varieties of diseases in which the results for 150 were excellent … The extensive clinical application of ear acupuncture in recent years shows that this simple method has multiple uses, attains speedy results, demonstrates efficacy, and is inexpensive.*

Diagnosis, treatment and prophylactic use

In modern China acupuncture is not merely used as treatment. When a doctor chooses herbal medicine[10] as a method, or is uncertain about a diagnosis, she may also use ear acupuncture as a diagnostic instrument.

In China both small and large surgical interventions are made when the patient is conscious. Acupuncture can give satisfactory alleviation of pain, for example in tooth extraction, but also in the performance of major operations in the abdomen or the thorax. When patients undergoing operations are given acupuncture anaesthetic instead of the conventional form, ear acupuncture is used, combined with body acupuncture, often with needles that are electrically stimulated. Ear acupuncture has shown itself to be an important component in achieving maximum alleviation of pain and in inducing the relaxation needed in operations when the patient should not sleep.

Ear acupuncture in other countries

India

India, like China, has a medical system which is several thousand years old. Both Indian and Chinese medicine are holistic, which is to say they are built on a complete way of seeing things. Indian medicine is called Ayur Veda. The book *Succhi Veda* (The Art of Piercing with a Needle) was written around 500 BC. According to Ayur Veda expert Chandrashekhar Thakur (Wexu 1985), the *Succhi Veda* gives an overview of how the ear may be used for diagnosis and treatment. According to Thakur, the Indians knew of a greater number of points in the ear than the Chinese

---

[10] In TCM herbal medicine is the most common form of treatment, more common than acupuncture, for example. See Ch. 2, A brief look at traditional Chinese medicine (TCM).

of the same period and developed a whole system for the treatment of illness with just stimulation of the ear. Like the Chinese, the Indians compared the ear with the kidney. They described the ear as a lotus blossom. Asthma was treated at a point on the lobe of the ear and allergies at a point on the apex which Nogier was to describe more than 2000 years later. Thakur tells too of newborn children in India having their ears pierced, not for ornamentation but to stimulate vitality and give protection against illness. He says children can be protected from running a temperature and diarrhoea during teething by making a hole in the ear.

Greece and Egypt

Knowledge of ear acupuncture reached Greece and Egypt around 400 BC. Hippocrates, known as the father of medicine, practised on the Greek island of Kos. Among the treatments he described were those involving stimulation of points in the ear to treat sexual and menstruation problems. Hippocrates lived for four years in Egypt and told how doctors there treated impotence and believed that women might be less likely to conceive if points in the ear were stimulated (Schelderup 1974). In his book *About reproduction*, Hippocrates describes how those who have been cut in the ear may still enjoy sexual relations and ejaculate but that there will be smaller amounts of sperm and it will be sterile. Hippocrates also taught that rapists could be made impotent by burning a zone in the ear (Överbye 1988). Sometimes rings placed at specific points in the ear were used to fight pain and in wars pain from wounds was alleviated by treating the ear.

Ancient Arab culture

Knowledge that one could treat pain through the stimulation of specific parts of the ear was common in Arab countries. Persian medical journals preserved among texts from 200 BC describe how the ear should be burned to relieve sciatica. In the 16th and 18th centuries elementary knowledge of ear acupuncture was to be found in Arab folk medicine. Pain was treated using small copper rings placed at special points in the ear.

Europe

In the 16th century European traders from the East India Company brought home with them from China knowledge of acupuncture and even ear acupuncture. Missionaries too brought such knowledge back to Europe after serving in Asia. One who propagated knowledge of acupuncture in the West after serving in Japan and on the Indonesian island of Java was the Dutch Jesuit Fen Rhijne. The use of ear stimulation for patients suffering from back pain was discussed sporadically in clinical reports in Europe. For several hundred years in France and Italy sciatica had been treated by burning points in the ear. In the 17th century the Portuguese doctor Lusitanus recommended treatment for sciatica and hip pains by using moxa at certain points in the ear, and in 1717 the Italian doctor Valsalva in his book *De aura humana* described a part of the ear which might be pricked to relieve toothache.

Paul Nogier's pioneering discovery

Paul Nogier, born in 1908 in France's second city Lyon, developed modern ear acupuncture in the 1950s. He discovered the reflex system in which the body is reflected as an upside down projection in the ear with reflex points that can be used for diagnosis and treatment. He called such treatment *auriculothérapie* (in English 'auricular therapy') and went on to develop auricular medicine.[11]

In his youth Nogier trained as a civil engineer but in the third year of the course fell ill and broke off his studies. When he was well again, he chose instead to follow in his father's footsteps and become a doctor. His father taught at the medical faculty in Lyon. Paul Nogier studied medicine but also became familiar with acupuncture via the texts of Georges Soulié de Morant, one of the first teachers of acupuncture in Europe.

In the 1930s Nogier also became interested in homeopathy and the teachings of Samuel Hahnemann.[12] He had great success treating his patients with a combination of Western medicine, acupuncture and homeopathic medicine.

Nogier learned from his study of homeopathy to take into account even the most seemingly insignificant symptom when judging a patient's condition and found that even mild treatment can change the course taken by an illness. He was to use this knowledge and his ability to observe and find the connection between different symptoms when he began to develop ear acupuncture. In the 1940s Nogier also continued his studies of body acupuncture. He was curious as to the nature of the acupuncture points and wanted to find out what they actually were. Along with his brother, also a doctor, he constructed, among other things, electrical point detectors so he could better measure and examine the points. Here his training as a civil engineer was put to good use.

Nogier started the so-called GLEM group *(Groupe Lyonnais d'Etudes Medicales)*. GLEM was an association of like-minded medical practitioners and enabled them to share their experiences with one another. They were interested in acupuncture, homeopathy and chiropractic and at their meetings tested, discussed and evaluated different methods. Out of these discussions grew a new awareness of the possibilities of ear acupuncture.

Burn marks in the ear

In 1951 Nogier's interest in ear treatment grew with the discovery that several of his patients had scars in the same part of their ears. It transpired that they had consulted a so-called 'wise woman', Madame Barrin, for treatment for sciatica and described how they had been relieved of pain for varying periods after being burned in the ear with a small, red-hot instrument.[13] Nogier was allowed to sit in and watch when Madame Barrin treated her patients and became fascinated by the efficacy of such treatment.

A small, flat piece of iron with an oval hole a few millimetres across was pressed against the ear so that the hole covered a special point in the antihelix often used to treat sciatica. A red-hot iron was then placed in the hole so that the patient came away with an oval burn mark. Madame Barrin had been taught which point should be burned by her father, who in turn had learned the method from a Chinese mandarin.

---

[11] Auricular medicine is a further development of the simpler form of auricular therapy, or ear acupuncture. It makes use of more advanced technical equipment for both diagnosis and treatment. In this book, however, we are concerned only with auricular therapy.
[12] Hahneman (1755–1843), a German doctor, founded the science of homeopathy which builds on the principle that 'like cures like'. Homeopathic medicine is thought to be effective even when greatly diluted.
[13] According to Rubach (2001) some of the patients had been given the same treatment in Africa.

Nogier himself began treating some of his patients who suffered from sciatica, with good results, by burning this point in the ear. He understood that this particular point in the ear corresponded to the small of the back, or more specifically the fifth lumbar vertebra (which may often be involved in sciatic pain) and for the sacroiliac joint.[14] Based on the assumption that there is a link between sciatic pain and the sacroiliac joint, Nogier extrapolated that he had found a reflex point in the ear corresponding to that joint.

From the start Nogier simply did what he had learned from Madame Barrin: he burned his patients in their ears. Later he tried a less barbaric method: he inserted an acupuncture needle and discovered that this gentler treatment also had a good effect. So began modern ear acupuncture in Europe.

Reflex points

Nogier came to the conclusion that if there was a reflex point in the ear for the sacroiliac joint, it was reasonable to suppose that there would also be reference points in the ear for other parts of the body, perhaps for *all* bodily parts and functions. In the years that followed he systematically examined his patients' ears. When patients visited his surgery, he looked carefully at their ears and palpated them (examined them by pressing against the skin) with a spring-loaded instrument to find points that might be sore. He found nearly all his patients to be sore at one or more distinct points and drew a map showing where these sore points were found, noting their relation to the bodily pain complained of by the patient.

Auricular therapy

Nogier discovered a pattern. Those patients who experienced pain in a certain part of the body, for example the elbow, had a sore point in the corresponding part of the ear (a special point in the scaphoid fossa; see Ch. 6, The ear and its acupuncture points). Those that had problems with another organ, for example the large intestine, had a tender point on the another part of the ear, in this case the cymba concha (see Ch. 6, The ear and its acupuncture points). If the sore point was stimulated there would be a reaction in the particular organ that was malfunctioning, or in the part of the body that was in pain. If a patient experiencing pain in an elbow was pricked with a needle in the sore point in the scaphoid fossa, the pain in the elbow diminished. Similarly the intestine of a patient suffering from constipation would begin to function when the tender point on the cymba concha was treated. Auricular therapy was born.

In addition Nogier discovered that when all the reflex points were drawn to make a map of the ear, they combined to form a picture of a man lying upside down. The points corresponding to the head were to be found in the lobe of the ear and parts of the arm and leg in the upper section of the ear, while those representing the intestines were located in the concha. He called the phenomenon of the upside-down man 'the homunculus' or 'little man'.

To begin with, Nogier treated primarily pain in the back and arms and legs with auricular therapy. These parts of the body are simply and plainly depicted in the ear. Later he evolved the method of treatment to take in pains in other parts of the body and malfunctioning organs.

---

[14] The sacroiliac joint is the barely moveable joint at the base of the spine between the sacrum and ilium and associated ligaments.

International recognition

Nogier's theory was built on the idea that illness and harming of body parts leads to changes in the ear, which is to say they activate parts of the ear so that biologically active points[9] can be found. By stimulating these active points the body can be healed. He presented his discovery for the first time at a congress of French acupuncturists in 1956. His theory was published in Germany in 1957 and rapidly spread to other countries. In 1958 his article was translated into Chinese and comparisons were made to Chinese research into ear acupuncture.

Different point maps

The investigation that was made by the Nanking Army Ear Acupuncture Research Team at the end of the 1950s confirmed to a large degree Nogier's map of the ear. However, certain points and zones were seen by the Chinese as being in different places. As a result there are now two maps for ear acupuncture, one French, one Chinese, where most points are in agreement, but with certain notable exceptions, for example when it came to the points representing the legs, kidneys and the uterus.

There are also other differences between the French and the Chinese way of looking at auricular therapy. Nogier did not think in terms of meridians as practitioners do in Chinese medicine.[15] He saw his discovery purely and simply as a reflex theory (the upside-down man). Even when it came to ear acupuncture the Chinese thought in terms of meridians. They said that meridians were represented in the ear in the same way as muscles, bones, nerves and blood vessels and that they could be influenced by the use of ear acupuncture.

When Nogier discovered the points system in the ear, he christened it auricular therapy. He chose not to use the word acupuncture because he claimed auricular therapy was built according to a different theory, one concerning reflexes. The Chinese on the other hand chose to call this form of treatment 'ear acupuncture' and saw it as being a part of the whole practice of acupuncture.

From China to the USA

When China opened up to Western politicians and journalists in the 1970s, there was great interest in traditional Chinese medicine. During American President Richard Nixon's state visit to China in 1971, James Reston, a member of the press corps accompanying him, fell seriously ill with appendicitis. His appendix was removed and later the Chinese physicians eased his post-surgery abdominal pain with needles. Reston wrote about his experiences and his article caused a sensation when it was published, sparking great interest in both body and ear acupuncture in the USA.

Auricular therapy evolves into auricular medicine

Paul Nogier continued his exhaustive studies of the ear. Not only did he investigate tenderness in close to 200 points in the ear which he had discovered, he searched too for changed electrical resistance in these points, and for changes in the structure of the ear and variations in skin colour, trying to find out how they might relate to the illness suffered by the patient. Fifteen years after his discovery of the reflex

---

[15] Meridians are channels for the qi, or life force. According to TCM there are 14 meridians evenly divided throughout the body. See Ch. 2, A brief look at traditional Chinese medicine (TCM).

zone map, Paul Nogier along with his son Raphaël, who was also a doctor, supervised the evolution of auricular therapy into auricular medicine. Because auricular medicine is a technically advanced method making use of electrical instruments, magnetic fields and treatment with lasers, various frequencies and light and colour filters, Paul Nogier was able to make use of his earlier studies as a civil engineer.

Vascular automatic signal

In the 1960s Nogier experimented with diagnosis in which the ear was stimulated along with a simultaneous taking of the patient's pulse. With one hand he took the patient's pulse, with the other he probed the ear by putting pressure on different points. Sometimes too he radiated the ear with light. Nogier discovered that the quality of a patient's pulse changed when active zones in the ear were stimulated. First he called this auricular cardiac reflex (ACR). When he later discovered that the pulse changed involuntarily, not just with ear stimulation but also with tactile or electrical stimulation of several other parts of the body, he changed the name, describing the phenomenon as vascular automatic signal (VAS).[16] The measuring of VAS became an important part of auricular medicine. It takes a great deal of practice. In the case of regular ear acupuncture, or auricular therapy, it is not necessary to search for VAS.

This book concerns auricular therapy (regular ear acupuncture), not auricular medicine (involving more technical variations of ear stimulation).

Ear acupuncture in modern Europe

As described above, modern ear acupuncture developed in parallel in France and China in the 1950s. It was not until the 1980s that the method came into more widespread use in France. By this time it had also been launched and become popular in the USA. Knowledge of the ear's reflex zones travelled round the world and interest in ear acupuncture grew in many European countries where it has since become firmly established. According to Coutté[17] every tenth doctor in France uses ear acupuncture for diagnosis or treatment.

Paul Nogier died in 1996. His son Raphaël followed in his father's footsteps, developing auricular medicine and giving instruction in its use. In many European countries there are schools in which ear acupuncture is taught and most longer courses on body acupuncture includes instruction in ear acupuncture.

Acupuncture, including ear acupuncture, is a form of treatment that has become the subject of a great deal of interest in many parts of the world. Different rules apply in different countries as to who may or may not become an acupuncturist. In some countries an acupuncturist must be a qualified doctor, while for example in Sweden the rules are more relaxed. Here ear acupuncture is used as part of the treatment not just by those acupuncturists who have received instruction in TCM but also by those who have been educated in Western acupuncture, for example physiotherapists, nurses and midwives. There are also those who practise just ear acupuncture.

---

[16] The Auricular medicinal terminology VAS should not be confused with a scale used in Western medicine to measure the degree of pain, which is also often shortened to VAS, standing for visual analogue scale.

[17] Alain Coutté is a French X-ray specialist who, in close collaboration with first Paul and later Raphaël Nogier, teaches auricular medicine in Denmark, the country to which he later moved.

The World Health Organisation and acupuncture

Since 1982 the World Health Organisation (WHO) has worked to try to bring about a standardisation of international acupuncture terminology in naming meridians and acupuncture points. Before this, confusion often arose, with various countries, authors and acupuncture schools using different abbreviations or translations of acupuncture terms. WHO appointed a working group to standardise terminology and the names of the reflex points in ear acupuncture. The idea was to support research, instruction and documentation of treatment. The working group put forward a report at a meeting in Lyon in 1990 (WHO 1990). The parts of the ear were named and coded and the meeting resulted in the WHO recognising ear acupuncture as a valid method of diagnosis and treatment and publishing a report listing ear acupuncture points where there was general agreement as to their location and their effect.

A brief look at traditional Chinese medicine (TCM)

Ear acupuncture is a variant of the larger discipline of acupuncture. This has its roots in traditional Chinese medicine (TCM), of which it is, to this day, considered an integral part, and this is why this chapter is devoted to a look at the basic concepts of TCM.[1]

Traditional Chinese medicine has for several thousand years been the treatment of choice of a fourth of the world's population for its illnesses, aches and pains, bodily malfunctions and infections. TCM is practised today in China in tandem with Western medicine. The acupuncture available in Europe is most often given to ease pain and builds on a Western interpretation of how the body functions (see Ch. 5, Explanatory models for acupuncture). But nowadays practitioners of classic TCM may also be found in many European and American cities.

Traditional Chinese medicine is every bit as logical as Western medicine but builds on a different understanding of reality. TCM has for centuries made use of the same basic concepts.

TCM: not *just* acupuncture

The roots of Chinese medicine go back 4000–6000 years back in time. While acupuncture is the best known facet of Chinese medicine in the West, TCM is by no means *just* acupuncture. Chinese medicine makes great use of herbal remedies. TCM comprises herbal medicine and acupuncture but also Tai Ji, Qigong and Tui Na (see discussions later in this chapter).

---

[1] The reflex theory established by Paul Nogier is not based on TCM.

The word 'acupuncture' derives from the Latin words *acus* and *pungere*. *Acus* means 'needle', *pungere* 'to pierce'. For more than 2000 years, long before mankind began to mine metal, people in China made use of 'needles' — first of stone and bone, then of ceramic splinters and bamboo — in order to stimulate different points of the body. Later acupuncture needles were made of bronze, gold and silver. A full set of the nine different types of needle described in texts from the era has been found in a grave dating from 200 BC.

In acupuncture treatment needles are stuck into the skin at the acupuncture points. These lie along the so-called meridians, channels for the qi, or life force. There are 12 pairs of meridians equally divided between the left and right sides of the body, along with meridians along the body's centre line, one to the front, and another to the back. The meridians lie just a little below the surface of the skin. Many of them are named after the organs which they are thought to be related to, for example the liver meridian, the small intestine meridian and the spleen meridian.

The acupuncture points are situated along the meridians and are the places where contact most easily can be made with qi. In the acupuncture points the qi comes close to the surface of the skin, where it can be found with an electrical point detector.[2] There are 365 regular acupuncture points on the human body in addition to a number of other points, and around 200 points in the ear.

The aim of acupuncture according to TCM is to stimulate these points and thus influence the flow of energy.

Herbal medicine

The most common form of treatment in TCM is with herbal medicine. Books that are a thousand years old describe how different herbs influence the internal organs and the energy channels connected to them. A herb can 'warm the lung's yin', 'strengthen the kidney's yang' or 'spread the lung's qi'. Herbs can be eaten in the form of tablets, boiled and drunk as tea, or inhaled or rubbed onto the body as lotion. Herbal medicines are not just made from parts of plants. They may also contain certain dried animal parts. The simplest form of herbal medicine is the food we eat. In China there has long been a strong awareness of how food, herbs and lifestyle influence our internal organs.

Tai Ji, Qi Gong and Tui Na

Tai Ji is a slow, meditative form of gymnastics whose aim is to benefit health by activating the flow of energy in the body. Tai Ji should be performed daily, preferably with a group of people (see Fig. 2.1). Qi Gong is still more meditative and less gymnastic. The aim is to correct the flow of energy and Qi Gong is in China used as a treatment for illness, for example in cases of asthma, allergy or cancer. Both Tai Ji and Qi Gong have become established in the West.

Tui Na is a manual treatment, best described as a mixture of Western massage, Japanese shiatsu (a form of massage of the acupuncture points and meridians), naprapathy and chiropractic.

---

[2] Body points are easily located with a point detector, at any time. The reflex points in the ear are only active and possible to find when there is something wrong with the corresponding part of the body.

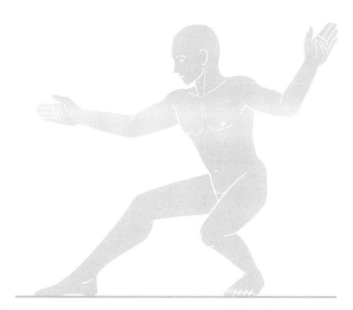

Figure 2.1 Tai Ji.

Moxa burning

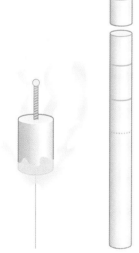

In Chinese medicine moxa burning is considered to be a part of acupuncture treatment. Moxa is a herb — a member of the same family as mugwort (*Artemisia vulgaris*) — which is regularly used in traditional Chinese medicine. In China moxa is so intimately linked to acupuncture that the written Chinese character for acupuncture actually means 'acupuncture and moxa burning'. Moxa in the form of a stick resembling a cigar can be burned over an acupuncture point in order to warm it. Or a 1-cm long piece of such stick can be placed on the end of an acupuncture needle and lighted (see Figs 2.2 and 2.3). The idea is that heat is conducted from the needle into the body. The essential oil from moxa will also cover the skin in a thin layer. Another method of treatment is for the herb in its natural form to be burned in a special moxa box containing a metal grill on which the glowing moxa rests a few centimetres above the skin. Sometimes too the skin may be deliberately burned with a small cone of moxa, in which case a small scar results.

Western acupuncturists use moxa less often than their Chinese counterparts. Treating with moxa requires a steady hand and takes time. In addition the smell of the herb can be penetrating and intense. Neither is the method scientifically proven. However, for TCM-educated acupuncturists, moxa remains an important part of the treatment.

Ear acupuncture makes less use of moxa. Moxa sticks are too thick to warm the small points of the ear and instead heat the entire ear. However, sometimes a much thinner stick, or 'tiger warmer', may be used to warm a specific point in the ear (see Ch. 9, Equipment and Ch. 11, Method).

Figure 2.2 and 2.3 A moxa cigar and burning moxa on needle.

Bleeding technique

Another technique involves making a point bleed. While in the old days acupuncturists would utilise a thick, triangular needle with sharp edges; today they would more often use a lancet (more commonly used to take blood samples), or perhaps a thicker needle to induce the flow of a few drops of blood. Both moxa burning and the technique of bleeding points in the ear are described in ancient Chinese texts. Bleeding may also be recommended in more modern books (see Ch. 9, Equipment and Ch. 11, Method).

Cupping

In China cupping is also a part of acupuncture treatment. Cups made of glass or bamboo are fixed to the skin after sucking out the oxygen in the cup to create a vacuum (see Fig. 2.4). Because a flat surface is needed, the technique is not used in ear acupuncture.

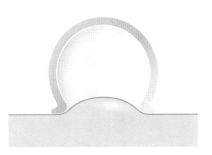

Figure 2.4 Cupping.

Differences between Western medicine and TCM

In Western schools of medicine parts of the body are judged and treated separately. Hospitals have specialised units: one for the heart; another for the kidneys; yet another for, say, cardiovascular surgery. TCM is holistic, meaning the body is treated as a whole. Things have to be seen in the wider context. Each part of the body is seen as a reflection of this wider context. A particular body part is interesting only in relation to the whole body, and the body must also be seen as intimately connected with the soul or spirit and the surroundings in which the patient lives before a doctor of TCM can understand how an illness has arisen and how it should be treated.

Qi

Qi is a basic concept in TCM. The nearest translation we have is 'life energy'. Qi is what distinguishes the living from the dead. The Chinese have been less concerned with what qi actually is, more with what it *does*. Qi makes it possible for everything to work and for renewal and transformation to take place. Acupuncture is a means of controlling the flow of qi.

Qi does not stand still in a reservoir in the body. It flows, circulating through channels, the so-called meridians. As long as the qi flows smoothly as it should, we remain healthy and able to resist illness. We become ill when there is a disturbance of the flow of qi, when there is too little or too much qi or when the polarity between yin and yang (see below) is unbalanced. All diagnosis in TCM is aimed at locating such stagnation and imbalance and the purpose of all treatment is to restore the flow of energy.

Yin and yang

Yin and yang are two polarities, two contrasting poles of energy. Everything in the universe may be divided into yin and yang. But all this is relative, meaning that yin and yang are not definitive descriptions or absolute concepts. One cannot often apply a label 'yin' or 'yang' because something may be yin in relation to one thing, yang in relation to something else. For example black tea is yang in relation to herbal tea but yin in relation to coffee. Yin can also become yang and vice versa. For example high temperature, which is yang, may turn into shivering, which is yin.

While they are opposites, yin and yang are dependent on each other for their existence and continuation: 'night' can only exist in contrast with 'day', 'cold' with 'hot'. Everything in the universe, including bodily organs and illnesses can be defined in terms on yin and yang.

A few examples of yin and yang division:

yin	yang
night	day
cold	hot
damp	dry
deep	shallow
nurturing	creative
inward	outgoing
female	male

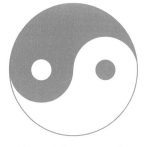

Figure 2.5 The symbol Tao.

The Tao symbol (Fig. 2.5) is a picture of yin and yang, showing them to be two parts of the same whole. The symbol portrays the ideal condition of perfect balance: yin and yang are the same size, there is no clearly defined border between them, they are part of a dynamic process where they can transform into each other and each one contains a part of the other.

Diagnosis

The starting point for diagnosis according to TCM is to locate the energetic disturbance in the energy field that gives rise to the symptoms the patient displays. The disturb-ance may then be treated with herbs, acupuncture, Tai Ji, Qi Gong or Tui Na. The Chinese doctor seeks a 'pattern in the fabric' and chooses a treatment that favourably influences that pattern.

The doctor begins by asking the patient about the symptoms, asking many more and very different questions to those that would be asked by a Western doctor. For example there may be detailed questions on possible perspiration, feelings of warmth or cold, on the patient's evacuation of urine and excrement and, in the case of female patients who are fertile, on their menstruation, even if the patient's illness might be seen by Western medicine as having no connection with such matters. The doctor is seeking a pattern in the balance between yin and yang, is using such information to make sense of a puzzle in order to gain an overview of how the various organs are working together and of the flow of energy in the meridians.

Tongue diagnosis

After questioning, the doctor looks at the patient's tongue. Tongue diagnosis has played an important part in TCM for thousands of years. The doctor looks at the tongue's colour, shape, coating, cracks and spots, and how it moves. There are zones on the tongue which correspond to the body's internal organs. The condition of the tongue's surface, cracks, colour changes and spots reveal, among other things, stagnation, weakness and where there may be excess heat, or yang. (See Fig. 2.6.)

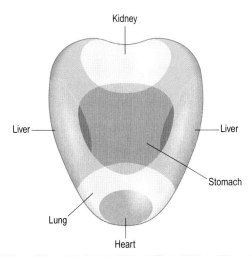

Figure 2.6 The tongue.

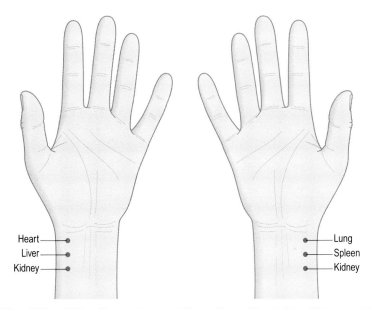

Figure 2.7 Pulse diagnosis.

Pulse diagnosis

When the doctor has examined the tongue, it is time for pulse diagnosis. The patient stretches out her wrists or lays them on a small cushion on the table. The doctor will use three fingers to take the patient's pulse at three positions on each wrist, using first gentle then stronger pressure to feel in depth. The quality of the pulse is judged according to 28 variables. Each pulse position is seen as corresponding to a certain organ and that organ's status can be monitored by the quality of the pulse at that position. (See Fig. 2.7.)

Ear diagnosis

Sometimes there will also be an examination of the ear, which will be inspected and palpated. The doctor looks for changes in colour, form and for possible sore points or points with a changed electrical resistance.[3]

Individual treatment

When the doctor has examined the patient, he will give advice concerning changes in diet or lifestyle, decide what treatment is suitable, which herbs the patient should take or what sort of acupuncture should be given (both body and ear acupuncture are considered). Three patients with the same symptoms, for example headache, can be given different treatments if the doctor decides that their problems have a different cause or 'root'. On the other hand, three patients with different symptoms (for example, migraine, high blood pressure and premenstrual tension) may be given the same treatment if the doctor decides that the 'root' of their troubles is the same ('the qi in the liver has stagnated') despite the fact that the three imbalances are manifested in completely different symptoms in each of the three patients.

Treatment is not standardised. In the West people with the same background and constitution but with the same symptoms (for example stomach ache with heartburn) might be given the same medicine (for example omeprazole) and the same dosage. So too in Western acupuncture patients with the same symptoms will most often receive the same treatment of the same acupuncture points. A TCM doctor, on the other hand, will choose herbs and acupuncture points to cater for each individual patient's needs and will reassess the treatment each time he meets the patient. The herbs and acupuncture points may be changed several times in the course of the treatment, as the patient's symptoms change.[4]

De qi

In Chinese acupuncture the aim is to achieve 'de qi', or 'needle sensation'. 'De qi' may be felt as a numbness, or a prickling, as if it is bubbling or flowing, but should not be experienced as strong pain. The needles can be stimulated by the acupuncturist rotating them a few times during treatment so that the 'de qi' feeling becomes more apparent. In Chinese acupuncture 'de qi' is intimately linked with the result. In other countries, for example Japan, there is a different needle technique, often with a sharper, smoother type of needle and there is no striving to locate 'de qi'. In ear acupuncture needles are not stimulated as a rule.

Many ear acupuncture patients find that the ear feels warm during treatment. This is also a form of 'de qi'.

---

[3] For more on ear diagnosis, see Ch. 10, Examination of the ear.
[4] NADA acupuncture, a standardised form of ear acupuncture used to treat people with a drug addiction, differs in that the same points are used in each treatment. See Ch. 13, NADA — using ear acupuncture to fight addiction.

Differences between ear and body acupuncture

The word 'acupuncture' derives from the Latin words *acus* and *pungere*. *Acus* means 'needle', *pungere*, 'to pierce'. Ear acupuncture and body acupuncture are two forms of treatment that resemble one another in that both involve pricking the skin with needles. To the uninitiated Westerner, the techniques in body and ear acupuncture may seem, to a large degree, the same. Impulses from acupuncture needles influence the nervous system and, no matter whether the needle is placed in the ear or the body, neurotransmitters and hormones are influenced in a similar way. However, there are certain clear differences between the two forms of acupuncture. We shall look at some of the most obvious of these in this chapter.

Historic differences

Traditional Chinese medicine (TCM; see Ch. 1, The history of ear acupuncture, and Ch. 2, A brief look at traditional Chinese medicine), of which body acupuncture forms a part, is thousands of years old. However, the acupuncturists of ancient China knew of only a few ear acupuncture points and had no idea as to the system in which they were arranged. Seen from a historical perspective, ear acupuncture in the form described in this book is a relatively new phenomenon, a reflex science developed in the 1950s.

Diagnostic differences

Active points

Body acupuncture points are always measurable at the same place. Draw an electrical point detector over the skin and it will give an indication of all the acupuncture points on the body, whether the person being examined is healthy or sick. The points on the body are always measurable because they are a part of the constant flow of energy in the meridians. This is not the case with the points in the ear. They are either 'on' or 'off'. Ear acupuncture points may be measured with a point detector only when they are 'on', which is to say when they are active because there is something wrong with the corresponding part of the body. Ear acupuncture is a reflex science: each part of the body has a point or zone in the ear where a malfunction in the corresponding body part registers. This malfunction may then be treated. A completely healthy human being in perfect balance should have no active points in the ear. (There are a few exceptions to this rule. Some so called masterpoints can be found with an electrical point detector even on a healthy person. See Ch. 6, The Ear: its parts and acupuncture points.)

Differential diagnosis

Because the points in the ear are active only when there is something wrong in the corresponding organ, an examination of the ear can be used either to confirm or rule out a diagnosis. The research team from Nanking cites acute abdominal pain as an example in their book (Huang 1974). If pain and other symptoms are atypical, making the diagnosis uncertain, the team says that, by searching in the ear for active points, the examining doctor can decide with a considerable degree of certainty if the cause of pain in the patient is a cyst on the ovary, a kidney stone, an inflamed appendix or a gallstone.

Taking the pulse

An important part of any examination by a TCM doctor is the taking of the pulse at different points on both wrists (see Ch. 2, A brief look at traditional Chinese medicine). In TCM, the condition of the various internal organs are 'read' in the quality of the pulse. While ear acupuncturists working with auricular medicine[1] will take the pulse of the patient during an examination, they will be looking for a completely different phenomenon, known as vascular autonomic signal (VAS; Ch. 1, The history of ear acupuncture). Nogier discovered that when active zones in the ear were touched or radiated with light, the patient's pulse changed. (In auricular therapy, the form of ear acupuncture described in this book, the pulse is *not* taken during examination.)

Other techniques

Semi-permanent needles

Body acupuncture makes use of acupuncture needles that stay in place for 20–40 minutes. In the ear one may use the same technique but semi-permanent needles may also be used. These remain in place, stimulating the acupuncture point for several days. In ear acupuncture this technique has been found to be effective for up to 2–3 weeks. Semi-permanent needles are used only in the ear.

---

[1]Auricular medicine is a developed and more technical form of regular ear acupuncture, auricular therapy.

Pellets

It is also possible to treat the ear without pricking it with a needle. A small metal pellet or a little seed is taped with band-aid to a specific point in the ear. The pellet or seed puts pressure on the point, generating what is known as acupressure. This can be a good alternative for patients with a fear of needles, with a blood infection or who may be too young for acupuncture. Pellets are often used in the ear, but only exceptionally on the rest of the body (see Su Jok, Ch. 4, Other microsystems).

Technical equipment

A skilled body acupuncturist needs no point detector or other electrical apparatus to find acupuncture points. The points can be located by measuring the distance to fixed 'landmarks' such as joints and other features of the skeleton. The body's acupuncture points are always at the same place.

In the ear the points are extremely close together. In ear acupuncture only active points are treated, so it's important to locate them correctly. The acupuncturist may make use of a mechanical point detector, or a pressure feeler, but many choose to equip themselves with an electrical point detector for still greater precision.

If, after your studies in auricular therapy (the regular ear acupuncture described in this book), you decide to go on and learn auricular medicine, this will entail the use of more advanced technical instruments, for example laser equipment.

Differing ideas concerning energy

The meridians

The TCM concept of body acupuncture is based on acceptance of a belief that there are energy channels — the meridians — which permeate the body in a fixed pattern. The acupuncture points lie along these. An acupuncture point is a place on the meridian where it is easier to reach the energy and influence it by puncturing, warming or massaging the point. Chinese literature on acupuncture takes it for granted that the meridians are also represented in the ear and that a stagnation[2] in a meridian can give rise to an active point in the part of the ear corresponding to the part of the body in which the meridian is located.

According to Paul Nogier (the French doctor who discovered auricular therapy), there are around 180 acupuncture points in the ear. These may be either reflex points (a reflection of a part of the body) or functional points (stimulation of the point influences a definite function). Nogier had a Western mind set. He saw the body's structure (skeleton, muscles, etc.) as being pictured in the ear, but did not recognise meridians. Neither did he describe acupuncture in terms of qi (the energy which the Chinese say flows through the meridians), or yin and yang, two other central concepts in Chinese medicine.

De qi

'De qi', the feeling around the needle which is sought after in body acupuncture — and regarded as being crucially important in achieving a good result — is not to be

---

[2]Stagnation of energy is the opposite to a free flow of energy.

found in the same way in ear acupuncture. In body acupuncture the acupuncturist stimulates the needles by rotating or moving them in such a way that the patient experiences feelings of tickling, pressure or radiation around the needle. It is this feeling that is called 'de qi'. In ear acupuncture the patient may experience a needle insertion as painful for a few seconds (particularly if semi-permanent needles are used), but once the needle is in place, the patient seldom has a clear feeling of it being there. Only exceptionally is there any discomfort.

In treatment of the ear with regular acupuncture needles, the patient may sometimes experience the feeling that the ear has become larger and warmer than usual. The ear may also redden. Such phenomena may be described as 'de qi'. However, contrary to body acupuncture practice, in ear acupuncture needles are not stimulated to generate the feeling.

Advantages for the acupuncturist

It takes a long time to learn body acupuncture. Several years of study are necessary in order to understand the classic Chinese system. Ear acupuncture is built on simpler foundations. Because the reflex points in the ear are divided into zones corresponding to the upside-down figure of a man, it is possible to learn the fundamentals in a few days. This means that a course in ear acupuncture is considerably cheaper than that for body acupuncture.

Saving time

It does not take a great deal of time to place needles in the ear. The patient can sit during treatment and need not get undressed. If semi-permanent needles are to be used, the patient need only remain in the clinic for the time needed for examination and the insertion of the needles. Body acupuncture takes much longer. The patient must undress, lie down and be cushioned with pillows and blankets. The needles stay in for 20–40 minutes and are stimulated several times during treatment. When the treatment is finished, the patient must get dressed again. All this takes time.

If the body acupuncturist needs to make use of points on both sides of the body, the session will have to be divided into two stages. As a result the patient must change position halfway through and treatment takes even longer. In ear acupuncture points corresponding to both sides of the body can be treated at the same time. This saves time both for the patient and the acupuncturist.

Group treatment

Ear acupuncture can, especially in cases of treatment for drug addiction, withdrawal symptoms or stress, be given to a group of people. This makes it extremely cost effective. Both time and space are saved in treating a group of sitting, fully dressed patients.

Another advantage of group treatment is that it can be less stressful for patients with high anxiety.

In ear acupuncture the patient can move during treatment. In body acupuncture the patient must lie still for 20–40 minutes. Ear acupuncture allows patients who may be worried and filled with anxiety, or may be in such pain that they cannot lie still for long periods, to experience more easily the benefits of acupuncture.

An ear acupuncturist can give several such group sessions an hour. (If you are making use of a standardised form of ear acupuncture such as NADA, 20 or so persons may be treated per hour. See Ch. 13, NADA – using ear acupuncture to fight addiction in the beginning….) Often existing premises such as an ordinary room in a house or office, a waiting room or a dining room can be used. No expensive and bulky examination benches are needed.

Ear acupuncture can be administered in simplified forms. The Nanking Army Ear Acupuncture Research Team summed this up in the 1960s: 'Whether indoors, outdoors, in open field, factory workshop, battlefield, trenches or classroom, ear acupuncture can be applied'.

Making it easier for the patient

Local points

It is commonplace in body acupuncture to make use of 'local points', i.e. points in the area where the pain is located. An advantage of ear acupuncture is that you can, without pricking the part of the body that is in pain, effect it in a positive way by pricking the corresponding part of the ear. Acupuncture points in the ear may even be used to treat parts of the body that may be 'off-limits' for the body acupuncturist, for example because they are in plaster, badly swollen or causing severe pain.

Two complementary treatments

Ear acupuncture and body acupuncture can be used separately or in combination. Ear acupuncture can be an excellent complement to body acupuncture.

The body acupuncturist can improve on results by making use of ear acupuncture both to treat the points in the ear corresponding to the organs or body parts that need treatment and to reduce stress and muscular tension in the patient.

However, ear acupuncture need not be administered in conjunction with body acupuncture. It can be the only form of acupuncture treatment.

Who can benefit from ear acupuncture?

In addition to patients, many health care professionals may have use for ear acupuncture:

- Body acupuncturists can add a good many more acupuncture points to their repertoire and gain a complement to the form of acupuncture they already practise.

- Chiropractors, osteopaths and naprapaths can use ear acupuncture as a means of getting muscles to relax, making — to take one example — spinal manipulation far easier. If ear acupuncture is given to relieve pain, deep trigger point massage may be possible on a patient who might otherwise be in no condition to tolerate this painful but extremely beneficial form of massage.

- Dentists can make use of ear acupuncture both as a form of anaesthetic and to calm otherwise anxious patients. Patients in a truly calm state can withstand a higher pain threshold.

- Doctors, nurses and midwives may find ear acupuncture an effective solution in alleviating pain, in aiding diagnosis and as a treatment for many different conditions.

■ Continued

- Various professionals working with patients who have alcohol or drug addiction problems can use ear acupuncture as an aid both during withdrawal and in the long rehabilitation phase, in which it can prevent relapse. It may also be used as treatment in the event of relapse.

- Therapists who treat stress, exhaustion, depression, patients with a high level of anxiety or with sleeping problems, can make successful use of ear acupuncture.

- Physiotherapists often find ear acupuncture an excellent complement to other methods and treatments for easing pain.

- Psychologists and psychotherapists can use ear acupuncture as an aid in getting patients to calm down and focus, and become more open to therapy, cutting down consultation times.

- Reflexologists, already working in a science concerning reflex zones, can profit by learning a new one.

Other microsystems

In the 1950s Nogier discovered that the ear contained a projection of the whole body turned upside down (see Fig. 4.1 and Ch. 1, The history of ear acupuncture). He described the phenomenon in his book *The Man in the Ear*, in which he likened the human being to a hologram. He named the phenomenon of projection of the whole in a certain part of the body 'somatotopie'. The word derives from the Greek, *soma* meaning 'body' and *topi*, 'topography'. In ear acupuncture we use the somatotopic map of the ear. There are many more somatotopies or microsystems in other parts of the body, grounded on the same basic idea: that the whole of the body may be reflected in one part of it.

Somatotopic maps and microsystems

The brain contains a systematic representation of the body in neurones in the cerebral cortex, in the subcortical thalamus and in the reticular formation system, an important reflex centre in the brainstem. Here the body is not reflected in the same proportions as in the actual body, so for example on the 'map' in the cerebral cortex the tongue and the hand are reflected in larger-than-life proportions (see Fig. 4.2).

In ear acupuncture the reflex points that correspond with parts of the body are divided up according to a systematic anatomical arrangement. The head and the hand occupy a larger area than they would if they were in proportion, while the thigh bone and the upper arm occupy a small space in the ear, precisely as in the somatotopic map of the brain. 'As with the somatotopic map in the brain, the auricular homunculus devotes a proportionally larger area to the head and hand than to the other parts of the body. The size of a somatotopic area is related to its functional importance, rather than its actual physical size' writes Terry Oleson (2003).

In the 1990s Dr Ralph Alan Dale, USA, maintained that it is not only in the ear that the whole body is represented. Corresponding microsystems with active points that can be used for diagnosis and treatment are also to be found in other parts of the body. Oleson

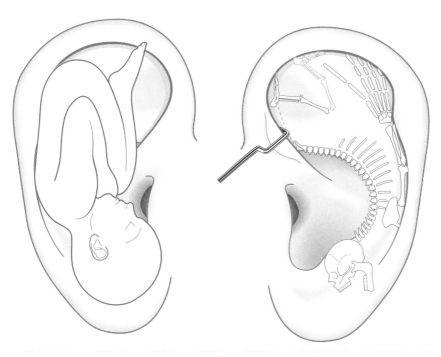

Figure 4.1 'The man in the ear'. The figure of a man projected in the ear.

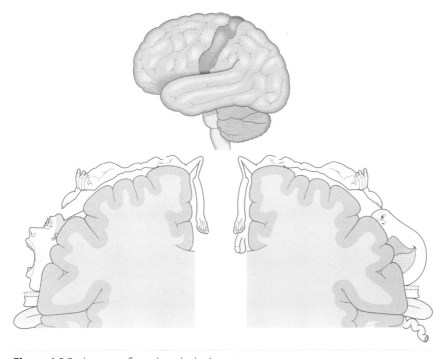

Figure 4.2 Body parts reflected on the brain cortex.

(2003) writes: 'Every micro-acupuncture system contains a distribution of acupoints that replicate the anatomy of the whole organism. Micro-acupuncture systems have been identified by Dale on the ear, foot, hand, scalp, face, nose, iris, teeth, tongue, wrist, abdomen, back and on every long bone of the body'.

In the following pages we shall look briefly at the best known of these other microsystems.

Reflexology

Reflexology was rediscovered at the beginning of the 20th century but had been used, according to Hagenmalm (2000), 5000 years ago in India and China. In the doctor's chamber in Saqqara in Egypt archaeologists have found a wall painting from 2330 BC showing doctors treating the soles of the feet (and the hands) of their patients with massage. According to the accompanying hieroglyphics, the doctor boasts: 'I shall treat you so that you sing my praises' (Hagenmalm 2000).

Reflexology is founded on the idea that the body's organs and parts are to be found outlined in a specific pattern on the underside of the foot (see Fig. 4.3). Reflexologists massage the soles of the feet with their fingers or with a soft rounded wooden implement. In the event of a bodily dysfunction, crystals build up in these

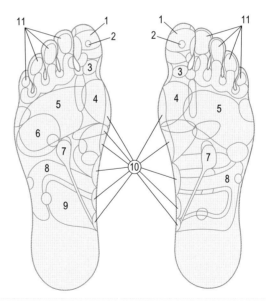

Figure 4.3 Zones on the underside of the foot that correspond to bodily organs:

1. Brain
2. Neck
3. Thyroid
4. Thyroid
5. Lung
6. Liver
7. Kidney
8. Large intestine
9. Small intestine
10. Spine
11. Sinus

zones, making them tender. This indicates that the corresponding organ is damaged in some way. The reflexologist examines these zones, makes a diagnosis and then treats the part of the body that is out of order by massaging the zone in question.

Su Jok

In Su Jok therapy the hands and feet are used to diagnose and treat illness. (*Su* means hand, and *Jok* means foot.) Jae Woo Park, a Korean professor,[1] discovered in the 1970s that the whole human being is represented both on the flat of the hand and the underside of the foot. His system is reminiscent of reflexology but the body parts have a different placing, and Su Jok includes several methods for stimulating active zones. Park made use of concepts from traditional Chinese medicine (TCM, see Ch. 2, A brief look at traditional Chinese medicine) in developing his method, among others qi (life energy) and meridians (the channels that transport qi)[2]. He also used concepts from ayur veda — Indian holistic medicine which has roots going back thousands of years — for example 'chakra' (energy centres).

In Su Jok the active zones of the hands and feet are stimulated with needles and pressure from pressure pens,[3] heat from moxa,[4] with light or by taping seeds or magnets over the point. In a more advanced form of Su Jok not only the organs but also the meridians are represented in the hands and feet.

Su Jok is used to treat both physical and psychiatric problems. This method of treatment is commonly used in Russia but still relatively new in Western Europe. They may either be used by therapists or by patients treating themselves.

In other schools a technique is taught in which one of the bones in the hand (the second meta-carpal) is stimulated to treat the entire locomotor system.

Korean hand therapy and acupuncture

Korean hand therapy and acupuncture, generally shortened to KHA (also KHT, Korean hand therapy), is a method reminiscent of Su Jok. It is founded on the same principle: that the body's parts and organs, along with the meridians, are to be found represented in the hand (see Fig. 4.4). Like Su Jok, KHA was developed in the 1970s, by Dr Tae-Woo Yoo. Since then KHA has been used to treat 1.5 million patients in South Korea and has spread to Japan, USA and Germany.

In KHA the positions of the various zones in the hand are different from those in Su Jok. The head, neck and backbone are seen as being represented by the middle finger, whereas in Su Jok the same body parts are depicted on the thumb.

Iris diagnosis

The Swedish priest and homeopath N. Liljequist, born 1851, wrote two books on how he discovered changes in the eyes of people with different illnesses or who

---

[1] Jae Woo Park first published his system in 1987.
[2] According to TCM there are 12 regular meridians, plus additional ones, running through the body.
[3] A pen-like object with a rounded point which puts pressure on the skin when examining or treating a point, i.e. palpating it. See Chapter 9, Equipment.
[4] Moxa is a herb used to warm the skin. See Chapter 2, A brief look at traditional Chinese medicine (TCM).

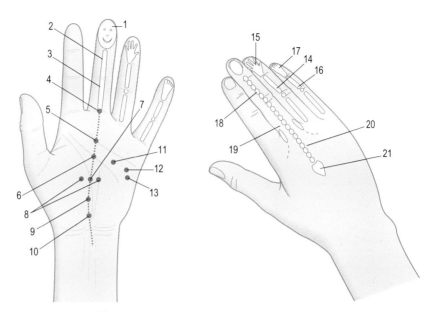

Figure 4.4 According to KHA the body is reflected in the hand in the following fashion:

1. Face	8. Ovaries	15. Hand
2. Throat	9. Bladder	16. Leg
3. Thorax	10. Sex organs	17. Foot
4. Heart	11. Kidney	18. Cervical vertebrae
5. Stomach	12. Large intestine	19. Thoracic vertebrae
6. Navel	13. Spleen	20. Lumbar vertebrae
7. Uterus	14. Arm	21. Sacrum

had been poisoned. He systematised his findings and published his first book on eye diagnosis in 1893 (Liljequist 1932). According to Liljequist, around the same time, the Hungarian doctor Ignaz Péczely noted similar changes in the eyes of his patients.

Homeopaths often use iris diagnosis. They can make a diagnosis by looking into a patient's eyes. The idea is that the body's various organs each have their place in the iris of the eye. If the organ is malfunctioning or has been damaged, there will be an indication of this in the iris in the zone allotted to the organ in question (see Fig. 4.5). If an arm is broken, immediately after the fracture there will be an indication in a certain part of the eye, and this indication will remain many years after the injury has healed. By discovering colour changes, spots or marks in different zones of the eye, the homeopath can see what has happened to the patient, which organ has been strained and perhaps also what is likely to happen as a result.

A TCM doctor will also look at the patient's eyes. In TCM the eye is thought to mirror 'shen' (the equivalent of 'soul' or 'spirit') so that the mental balance and strength can be read in the lustre of the patient's glance.

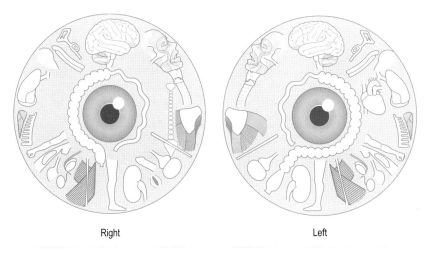

Right   Left

Figure 4.5 Specific areas of the iris change when the body's organs fail to work as they should.

Tongue diagnosis

A careful study of the tongue has for thousands of years been an important part of the examination in classic acupuncture. The various zones of the tongue are seen as corresponding to different organs, which is to say that the tongue too contains a microsystem (see Fig. 4.6). The doctor asks about the patient's symptoms, then studies the tongue very carefully, noting its colour, shape, coating, and whether there are any cracks and spots. The tip of the tongue corresponds to the heart, becoming red in the case of many heart-related illnesses. The side of the tongue represents the liver and when there is a malfunctioning of that organ it will often be covered in small spots. The central area of the tongue corresponds to the stomach and can be red, pale or have a deep crack, depending on the stomach disorder.

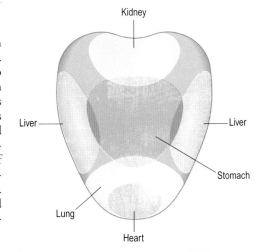

Figure 4.6 On the tongue there are zones which correspond to some of the body's internal organs.

Pulse diagnosis

Pulse diagnosis is based on another microsystem with internal organs represented on the wrists. Once the Chinese doctor has questioned the patient and looked at the tongue, it is time for pulse diagnosis. The patient stretches out his wrists or lays them on a small oblong rice cushion on the table. The doctor will use three fingers to take the patient's pulse at three positions on each wrist simultaneously, and will judge the pulse according to 28 variables (see Fig. 4.7). He will first use only light pressure against the patient's wrist, then increase it. The light pressure allows the doctor to check one specific organ, the increased pressure another one. Every organ's status can be monitored by the quality of the pulse. The doctor can, among

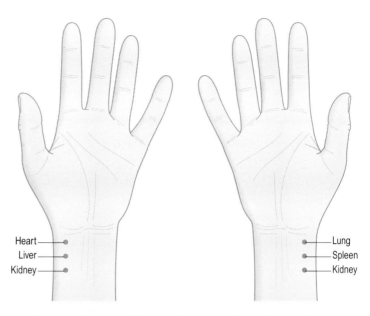

Figure 4.7 There are reflex zones for internal organs at three places on the wrist.

other things, feel if the organ lacks energy, or the energy has stagnated, if there is a lack of 'blood',[5] or if a pathogenic factor has invaded the organ.[6]

Scalp acupuncture

Head, or scalp, acupuncture was developed in China in the 1970s. The underlying idea is that on the scalp are zones representing arms and legs, the back, vasomotor zones, the optical area, the gastric area, the thorax, the motor area, speech, etc (see Fig. 4.8). The acupuncturist inserts long needles under the skin along the skull bone and stimulates them manually or with electricity. The symptoms most often treated are those that follow a stroke (lameness and speech difficulties) but also backache and other painful conditions, Parkinson's disease, Ménière's disease, headaches, dizziness, bedwetting, trigeminal neuralgia and asthma.

Wrist and ankle acupuncture

Wrist and ankle acupuncture, often shortened to WAA, was developed in the 1970s. The method comes from China, and like ear and skull acupuncture differs from methods of treatment in TCM. WAA is a reflex theory, based on the concept that the body is divided into six bilateral longitudinal zones (see Fig. 4.9). Needles

[5] 'Blood' in TCM is seen as being more than simply actual physical blood.
[6] In TCM external factors such as cold, heat and wind, along with emotional disturbances such as fear and sorrow are seen as factors that can cause illness by 'invading' the human being.

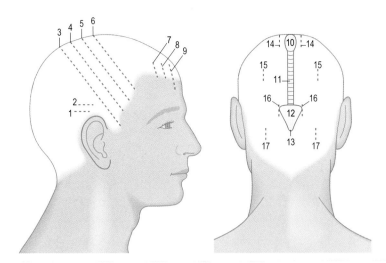

Figure 4.8 Zones treated with scalp acupuncture to aid different problems.

1. Speech zone
2. Dizziness and auditory zone
3. Sensory area
4. Motor area
5. Zone for shaking and trembling
6. Area that influences the width of blood vessels
7. Reproduction area
8. Stomach zone
9. Thoracic zone
10. Neck zone
11. Back zone
12. Sacral zone
13. Coccyx zone
14. Lower extremities zone
15. Speech zone
16. Sight zone
17. Balance zone

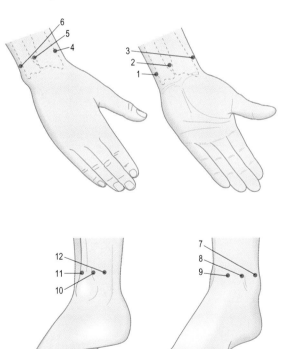

Figure 4.9 Six points/zones on the wrist and the same number on the ankle correspond with the rest of the body.

1. Upper 1
2. Upper 2
3. Upper 3
4. Upper 4
5. Upper 5
6. Upper 6
7. Lower 1
8. Lower 2
9. Lower 3
10. Lower 4
11. Lower 5
12. Lower 6

are inserted into the wrists and ankles in the zones that correspond to the parts of the body needing treatment. Only six acupuncture points are used on the wrist and six more on the ankle. (In TCM there are 365 regular acupuncture points.) In WAA the needles are inserted superficially and pulled under the skin. It also differs from TCM (in which needles can be inserted deeply) in that WAA does not strive to achieve 'de qi' — the characteristic feeling of numbness, pricking and similar, which according to TCM should occur in acupuncture. This means that WAA treatment is neither painful nor unpleasant. WAA can be used to treat both pain and other conditions.

5

Explanatory models for acupuncture

Chapter contents

The way acupuncture works may be described from various perspectives. Broadly speaking, such explanations are grounded either in Western classroom medical theory or in Asiatic theories concerned with energy, with which we are less familiar in the West. In Ch. 2, A brief look at traditional Chinese medicine (TCM), explanations of the effects of acupuncture were based on such ancient Chinese concepts as qi, yin and yang and stagnated energy.

This chapter summarises the effects of acupuncture as seen from a Western perspective with explanations grounded in neurophysiological and cellular biological theory. To qualify as scientific, explanatory models will be based on research, knowledge and well-tried practical experience.

In Sweden, where I practise acupuncture, the National Board of Health and Welfare *(Socialstyrelsen)* regards acupuncture as a scientific method comparable with other healthcare treatments.[1] However, it took time for acupuncture to reach such a point. There are still ambiguities as to exactly *how* acupuncture works. A huge problem in acupuncture research is that the discipline doesn't fit the only research model accepted in Western medicine. First therefore, we shall review the problems related to describing in a scientific way how acupuncture works. This will be followed by a summary of the way it works, verified by research … despite all these difficulties.

Research problems

In the Western medical world, in order for a method to be regarded as scientific, or for a hypothesis to be accepted, the method and its effects should be examined in at least one study — preferably more — that

---

[1] Swedish Socialstyrelsen memo 11/93.

follows an acceptable format. This format has been designed for the testing of medicine, which means studies that are randomised, controlled and double-blind. It should also be possible to repeat the test, which presupposes that therapists can follow exactly the same procedure with every treatment. Such a model for evaluation works well when used to test medicines, but creates difficulties for treatment methods that do not fit the format. Articles about such treatment methods won't be published in scientific medical journals and as a result will not be accepted in the medical world.

Acupuncture, along with massage, chiropractic, reflexology and psychotherapy, are examples of methods of treatment that don't fit the format for scientific validation required in medicine. The difficulty is that there is no good control method and tests cannot be made double-blind, because patients most often can guess whether or not they have received the 'right' treatment.

Randomised testing

In a trial two or more groups should be given different treatments. One can compare two or more methods of treatment with each other, or a presumably effective treatment with a placebo. Randomising means that the patients cannot choose which group they should be in. Patients who have agreed to take part in a study are randomised, put in one or the other group, by drawing lots. This is one of the easiest scientific criteria to fulfil in a study of acupuncture.

Controlled testing

In order for a study to be controlled, it is necessary to compare one treatment with another. When it comes to the testing of medicines, this is easy: one group of patients (the treatment group) is given tablets with an active medical substance and the control group is given placebo tablets without any known active ingredient (so-called sugar pills). The tablets containing the active medical substance and the placebo tablets can be made to appear identical and placed in similar packaging with a coded label. Only when the experiment is over is the label decoded and the evaluator learns who received what, active substance or placebo.

In all studies of acupuncture it is difficult to find a valid control method because, of course, patients know well whether or not they are being pricked with needles. To insert needles adjacent to the 'right' point in the control group would mean good acupuncture was being compared with bad, rather than that one patient was receiving acupuncture, the other not. Many of the effects of acupuncture are non-specific and a certain effect can be achieved even if the needle is inserted somewhere other than the 'right' point. (For example, the DNIC effect — diffuse noxious inhibitory control system, a bodily mechanism that alleviates pain — comes into play each time the skin is penetrated with a needle, such penetration being associated with pain.) Another problem specific to ear acupuncture is that the points are very close to one another (there are around 200 of them in the ear) and this means that one may prick another point if one tries to insert a needle a few millimetres away from the 'right' point. In addition, several closely adjacent 'points' in the ear might be better described as one 'zone' and here it is impossible to use a point a few millimetres from the 'right' point as a control.

Comparisons are sometimes made between acupuncture in which one produces 'de qi'[2] and another more superficial variant in which there is no needle stimulation to produce 'de qi'. However, this form of control cannot be used when it comes to ear acupuncture where the needles are not normally stimulated to bring about 'de qi' and in which all needles are placed on the surface. Besides, even when used to test body acupuncture, this is a dubious method of control because certain acupuncturists make use only of surface needle placement. In addition, a large part of the population may have been given acupuncture earlier in life, thus knowing what needle stimulation and 'de qi' should feel like. If such persons take part in the study and then receive acupuncture without experiencing 'de qi' they will in all likelihood suspect that they are part of the control group.

Double-blind testing

A test is said to be double-blind when neither the patient nor the person carrying out the treatment knows whether that treatment is genuine or placebo. Double-blind studies works well when it comes to testing medicines but when it is used to test many other methods of treatment it becomes untenable. An acupuncturist knows — hopefully! — if the point being treated is 'right' or 'wrong' and the patient is obviously aware of being pricked with a needle. Similarly, people receiving treatment by a chiropractor clearly feel whether their bones are being manipulated or not. There are also difficulties in double-blind testing of, for example, massage and psychotherapy.

Attempts have been made to carry out double-blind acupuncture studies by instructing personnel to give sham acupuncture so that they believe what they are doing is right when they practise the treatment on the control group. Not only is this unethical but there is always a risk that the same personnel, once the study is over, will continue to use sham acupuncture. Besides, the personnel concerned in testing need only to open a textbook on acupuncture to discover that they have been taught incorrectly.

If one cannot carry out a double-blind study, the next best thing is to arrange one that is single-blind. In a single-blind test the person carrying out the experiment knows whether the patient is being given genuine treatment or placebo, but the objective is that the patient remains unaware of it. In a single-blind study it is important that the person carrying out the test remains as neutral as possible and does not transmit his belief in the efficacy of the different treatments to the person being tested. However, if the person giving the treatment in the study succeeds in being completely neutral, the experimental situation will not be comparable with treatment in a clinic, where it is not only permissible but also desirable for personnel to be enthusiastic, personable, encouraging and supportive.

In studies which cannot be made double-blind it is important that the evaluator is 'blinded', that is does not know whether the patient has been given active treatment or placebo.

The irrelevance of animal experiments

A great part of medical research is carried out on animals. In a laboratory where acupuncture is used on rats, it is difficult to achieve a treatment situation comparable

---

[2] 'De qi' is a sensation produced by an acupuncture needle, a feeling that the qi, or energy, is moving. It can be experienced as a pressure, or as energy radiating or streaming beneath the skin.

with that of treatment of humans. The needles used in animal experiments are the same as those used on humans. Used on animals they are disproportionately large because the animals' bodies are so much smaller than those of human beings. A 0.3-mm thick needle used on a rat is the equivalent of a 6-mm thick needle used on a human. This results in a more painful insertion, causing the animal more stress. When pain and stress are generated, other mechanisms come into play. Thus the result of treatment on stressed rats, strapped to the test bench, is not comparable to acupuncture practised on relaxed, motivated human beings.

Difficulties of repetition

According to the accepted scientific evaluation format, it should always be possible to repeat a study. Thus the treatment should be precisely the same in each case for all patients. This means that individually tailored treatment such as the acupuncture practised in TCM, or ear acupuncture given to active points, will not fit the accepted format. What distinguishes TCM therapy is that the herbs or acupuncture points are decided upon individually for each patient and may be changed as the patient's condition changes. The ear acupuncturist may find that the active points change place from day to day, so that points to be treated may also have to be changed.

Problems with research on drug abusers and psychiatric patients

Difficulties with any scientific evaluation of acupuncture, as detailed above, become still greater when, as happens with research into NADA,[3] tests are carried out on people with drug addiction, alcohol problems, and psychiatric illnesses or even with double diagnosis. Such people are seldom as easy to direct or as devoted to the world of research as patients in a study of, say, sciatica or high blood pressure often are. If a study has a high drop-out rate it is thought to be less reliable. But if the people taking part in the experiment are actively psychotic, are drug abusers or homeless, it will be more difficult to motivate them and the drop-out rate is bound to be higher. While this is a predictable effect, it diminishes the credibility of the study from a scientific point of view, making it more difficult to get significant (statistically secure) variation between groups.

Quantitative and qualitative research

The greater part of the research which is published (and which thus constitutes the basis of what is regarded as truth in the medical world) is quantitative. This means that one measures, weighs or in some other way registers data which can be converted into tables and statistics. The larger the group of patients being examined, the more secure the result.

An alternative is to make use of qualitative research methods. This too is subject to strict rules but measures the result in another way. Qualitative research is based on the patient's experience and whether the treatment gives results. The examination can be based on interviews and the group of people undergoing experimentation need not be large. A great deal of research into nursing is carried out using qualitative studies, but in the medical world results gained in this way are not

---

[3] NADA is a standardised form of ear acupuncture given to treat addiction, see Ch. 13, NADA – using ear acupuncture to fight addiction in the beginning.

reckoned to be as scientifically valid as those obtained from quantitative research. Qualitative studies are still not published in most scientific medical journals. On the other hand, other working groups besides doctors — for example psychologists, sociologists and nurses have for decades had their own journals in which the status of qualitative research approaches that of quantitative research.

Using qualitative methods it is possible to make use of experience and treatment results missed by quantitative research. Qualitative evaluation can create an opening for the methods of treatment which hitherto have not been accorded scientific status because it has not been possible to evaluate them according to the format acceptable within quantitative medical research.

Evidence-based medicine and nursing

In recent years the concept of evidence-based medicine and nursing has gained ground in healthcare. Evidence should be grounded in experience collected from diverse sources. Evidence-based nursing means that the care should be grounded on the results of research, for example randomised, controlled, blind studies and meta-analyses,[4] but also on proven experience and on patients' experiences and wishes.

If one chooses a treatment method which has been subjected to less scientific evaluation, it is important that it should be safe (have few undesirable side effects), that the patient wants it and that it is cost effective.

Comprehensive acupuncture research

Despite the many difficulties encountered in the evaluation of acupuncture, in the past 25 years there have been a great many studies which, in different ways, have sought to examine certain effects of the discipline. The vast majority of these concern acupuncture as a means of alleviating pain. In recent years findings from research into the effect of acupuncture on many illnesses and dysfunctions have been published in scientific medical journals around the world. There are today (November 2007) 12.381 entries in the Medline database of scientific medical articles that contain the word 'acupuncture'. Most explanatory models used for body acupuncture also apply in principle to ear acupuncture.

A complicated process

There is no simple answer to the question of how acupuncture works. Many different mechanisms are involved. The human being is a complex biological phenomenon. Functions are governed by networks of nerve fibres working in collaboration with a myriad of chemical substances, hormones and enzymes. It has been shown clearly that acupuncture exerts an influence at many different levels, but there is, as yet, no complete picture of all the processes it sets in motion.

Because in many respects body and ear acupuncture work in the same way, we shall go on to examine first theories applying to both forms, and second theories devoted specifically to ear acupuncture.

---

[4] Meta-analysis is a compilation of data from several independent examinations.

The effects of acupuncture

In scientific studies it has been clearly shown that acupuncture relieves pain, boosts the body's immune defence system, regulates physiological imbalances and has a calming effect on patients.

Acupuncture as a painkiller

Most research shows that acupuncture relieves pain. Thousands of studies have documented the effect and researchers have also been able to explain the mechanism in which pain is alleviated in a scientifically acceptable way. We now know that many different factors contribute to the effect of pain relief.

Clinically, acupuncture is most often used in the Western world to relieve pain. Nowadays thousands of physiotherapists and midwives are given an abbreviated, Western training in acupuncture. Pain in the locomotor system (muscles and skeleton) is often treated with acupuncture and in Sweden and other European countries more and more maternity clinics offer acupuncture to women giving birth.

In cases of neurogenic (nerve) pain, however, acupuncture has a more uncertain effect.

Acupuncture can give such powerful pain relief that in certain cases operations may be performed without the patient having to be given an anaesthetic. In Asia acupuncture is used not only for minor surgical interventions, for instance the removal of a patient's tonsils, but also for major operations to the thorax and abdomen. When acupuncture is used instead of chemical anaesthetic, or in combination with it, ear acupuncture is always used, sometimes combined with body acupuncture, and usually with the needles electrically stimulated.

In most Western countries, no major surgery would be undertaken using acupuncture as a substitute for anaesthetic. However, it is becoming common — at least in Sweden — for midwives to sew up ruptures that occur during childbirth with no other anaesthetic than acupuncture.

The effect that acupuncture has in alleviating pain may be explained in several ways. It is well known that endorphins[5] are released during acupuncture. In addition to endorphins, many other neurotransmitters (the chemical messengers of the nervous system) and hormones (chemical substances released by glands into the blood, which influence other organs that have receptors for them) are released, which contribute to the pain relief. Another explanation may be that pain impulses are blocked at spinal cord level and don't reach the brain (gate control theory, see below).

It is often forgotten, however, that pain relief from acupuncture does not always depend on a neurological blocking or on an increase in the amount of endorphins. For example, ischaemic pain (due to lack of oxygen because the blood cannot circulate) is relieved by acupuncture because of its effect in dilating the blood vessels, while the painful effects of gastric ulcers are diminished because of acupuncture's effects in regulating the amount of hydrochloric acid secreted in the gastric juices.

---

[5] Endorphins are substances produced by the body that are sometimes referred to as the body's own morphine. There are more than 100 endorphins. During the early days of acupuncture in the West, a great deal of its effects were ascribed to the release of endorphins. Now we know that endorphins are released mostly as a result of strong stimulation (as used in experimental acupuncture) while, in the milder form of acupuncture more common in clinical praxis, other mechanisms come into play.

Boosting immune defence

Acupuncture influences the immune system favourably. The first known textbook on acupuncture (written before the birth of Christ) concerns treatment of illnesses with high temperature and indicates that the most common use of acupuncture at that time was as a treatment for infections. When acupuncture reached the West 2000 years later, it was for a long time seen as being merely a method of pain relief. Now Western research has confirmed that there is a relationship between the central nervous system and the hormonal system which makes it possible for the immune system to be influenced during acupuncture. According to research, acupuncture increases the number of natural killer (NK) cells, boosts the activity of such cells and has a favourable effect on immunoglobulins.

Regulating physiological imbalance

The ancient Chinese understanding was that acupuncture could be used to influence many different illnesses and somatic dysfunctions. In modern times this understanding has been confirmed by research. Studies have shown that acupuncture influences for example, the functioning of the heart, blood vessels, blood pressure, the ability to breathe, the body's hormonal balance, the stomach and the intestines, the composition of the blood and the urinary system.

Acupuncture is considered to be a balancing treatment, regulating both over- and under- bodily functioning. As a by-product of studies originally initiated to measure other acupuncture effects, we know that it can lower high blood pressure and raise low blood pressure. More research is necessary before we have a complete explanation as to how this happens, however.

The calming effect of acupuncture

Only in more recent times has the psychological effect of acupuncture received attention in the West. In studies made of sleeping habits, a majority of people suffering from disturbed sleep said that they slept better after acupuncture treatment. Acupuncture also has a calming, stress-reducing, antidepressant effect. This may, among other things, be a result of the effect acupuncture has on the adrenal gland. It may immediately affect production in the adrenal medulla of catecholamines.[6] It may also exert a slower effect on the adrenal cortex. During acupuncture there is a favourable effect on levels of, among other things, serotonin,[7] GABA,[8] oxytocin[9] and perhaps most important of all in cases of stress, cortisol.[10]

---

[6] The hormones adrenaline, noradrenaline and dopamine. Catecholamines are transmitter substances in the central and peripheral nervous system.

[7] A neurotransmitter which plays an important part in alleviating pain, the ability to sleep, our emotional state, aggression and appetite. Diminished levels of serotonin are thought to produce depression and increase the risk of suicide. Newer antidepressant medicines, such as selective serotonin reuptake inhibitors (SSRIs), the so-called 'happiness pills', help to resume production of serotonin.

[8] Gamma-aminobutyric acid, which has an inhibiting effect on the central nervous system. Insufficient levels of GABA can be a cause of worry, anxiety and neuromuscular diseases.

[9] Oxytocin is known as the 'feel well hormone'. It is important for lactation but is also released — to give two examples — when we laugh or are given massage.

[10] Cortisol is a stress hormone which has an important effect on, among other things, levels of sugar and insulin, and the body's defence against infections and allergies. In cases of long-term stress, the cortisol levels rise, which, among other things, has a negative influence on the ability to sleep, the walls of the blood vessels, the function of the pancreas, immune defence and production of abdominal fat.

The autonomous (visceral) nervous system, which controls visceral organs, consists of the sympathetic and parasympathetic nervous systems. The sympathetic system boosts the activity of the internal organs and prepares us for fight and flight. The parasympathetic system activates the digestive process and makes it possible for us to rest. The effect of body and ear acupuncture is to a large degree the same (calms the sympathetic activities and activates parasympathetic functions), though ear acupuncture exerts greater influence on the parasympathetic system than body acupuncture. This may explain why ear acupuncture is frequently used to treat anxiety, stress and disturbed sleep.

Reducing muscular tension

Ear acupuncture can bring about an immediate reduction in muscular tension. Many people who have been given acupuncture describe how their bodies feel relaxed afterwards. In the case of certain forms of body acupuncture, for example trigger point acupuncture, in which so-called trigger points in a muscle are stimulated, the muscle can very clearly relax even during stimulation. This happens because the motoneurones of the nervous system are influenced.

Various explanatory models

Acupuncture researchers in both China and the West have mapped out several of the ways in which acupuncture works. Many of them have studied how the neural pathways act as a conduit for the acupuncture impulses, others how acupuncture influences the release of different hormones and neurotransmitters. What is certain is that many different factors contribute to the effects of acupuncture.

What happens in the nervous system during acupuncture?

Many experiments have been carried out, primarily on animals but also on humans, to show which neural pathways act as conduits for acupuncture impulses. Researchers have studied where the switching occurs in the pathways and which chemical substances are released at the different switching stations on the impulse's journey from the point in which the needle has been inserted to the brain. Acupuncture has an influence at several levels in the nervous system. Factors that influence which mechanisms come into play include needle stimulation technique (whether painful or not), and the choice of acupuncture points (whether in the same segment as the part of the body that is in pain or in another segment). The effect of body and ear acupuncture is to a large degree the same, but ear acupuncture seems to influence the parasympathetic nervous system more than body acupuncture.

The influence on the sympathetic nervous system

When there is mild stimulation of the acupuncture needle, activity is inhibited in the sympathetic nervous system which is the part of the autonomous nervous system that prepares the body for fight. However, in painful stimulation of the acupuncture needles, as may be achieved, for example, by using strong electrical stimulation, the activity in the sympathetic nervous system increases.

Acupuncture influences the flow of blood in the body's tissue, both locally and in general. One can observe a reddening around the needle and many patients report feeling warm during treatment. This can depend on an inhibition of activity in the sympathetic nervous system.

If the goal is to diminish the patient's stress levels, it is important to give a mild acupuncture treatment, one that is not painful, so that activity in the sympathetic nervous system is reduced.

In ear acupuncture the acupuncturist searches for active points with a probe or a point detector which registers changes in electrical activity in some of the points of the ear (see Ch. 10, Examination of the ear and Ch. 9, Equipment). The increase of the conductive ability which the point detector registers in the skin between active and non-active points can be caused by the sympathetic nervous system innervating the sweat glands.

Changes in the surface of the ear that can sometimes be seen with the naked eye during ear diagnosis — for example pale spots or flaking skin — may be caused by blood vessels in that part of the ear contracting (see Ch. 10, Examination of the ear and Ch. 9, Equipment). This can, in turn, be caused by heightened activity in specific sympathetic nerves.

Activation of the HPA axis

In recent years the HPA axis has become a frequent talking point in research into stress. HPA is an acronym for hypothalamic pituitary adrenal,[11] and refers to a collaboration between the brain's hypothalamus which produces a releasing factor — a chemical messenger which initiates a process in the body — stimulating the pituitary gland to produce ACTH (adrenocorticotrophic hormone) which creates homeostasis in many bodily functions. In addition ACTH stimulates the adrenal gland to produce more or less of the stress hormone cortisol, which prepares the body to exert itself and has a strong anti-inflammatory effect. Stress increases the release of cortisol. Cortisol — cortisone in medicinal form — is beneficial in cases of inflammation, but high cortisol levels have many negative effects.

The stress relief effect produced by acupuncture can be a result of a modulation in the HPA axis. Levels of stress hormones such as ACTH and cortisol after acupuncture depend on the strength of the stimulation. The levels are heightened by painful acupuncture, in which needles are stimulated to a high intensity, but are lower under mild stimulation. The same is true of levels of adrenaline and noradrenaline. If the aim is to reduce stress in the patient, it is important to administer a mild acupuncture treatment that is not painful so that activity in the HPA axis is curtailed and the cortisol level declines.

What happens around the needle

When an acupuncture needle is stuck into the skin, there is a local reaction around the field of pricking point. The skin's receptors and nerve fibres are activated.

---

[11] The hypothalamus is a part of the brain's limbic system which plays a decisive role in the regulation of the autonomous nervous system. The pituitary lies in the midbrain and influences the entire inner secretion system by controlling the secretion of a large number of hormones. Adrenal in this case refers to the adrenal glands, which produce, among other things, cortisol.

Neurotransmitters are generally associated with the brain but even at a local level neuropeptides (chemical substances) are released. One example is CGRP (calcitonin gene-related peptide), which can dilate blood vessels and in low doses has a favourable local anti-inflammatory effect. Acupuncture results in a local increase in the circulation of blood and lymph. Other substances which are released around the needle are substance P,[12] bradykinin,[13] serotonin, endorphins, galanin, somatostatin[14] and VIP.[15] Some researchers say that electrical phenomena also occur around the needle.

What happens in the spinal cord

In the spinal cord impulses are sorted according to Gate Control Theory, which won Melzack and Wall a Nobel prize in 1967. Their research was welcomed by acupuncturists because it helped to explain acupuncture's pain-inhibiting effect. The theory applies to both body and ear acupuncture. In short it says that pain and acupuncture impulses are transported in different neural pathways. At spinal cord level the body chooses to let through only one of these sequences of impulses. It is a bit like a railway tunnel where only one train at a time may pass. The train that acupuncture uses always gets priority, which means that the train being used by pain, travelling on another track, is stopped, at least for a short time. Pain is thus stopped in the spinal cord and never becomes conscious. Dynorphin and enkephalin are also involved in gate control.

Gate control theory has often been used to explain the effects of acupuncture. However, it goes only part of the way towards accounting for the fact that acupuncture can take away pain for a long time, sometimes several weeks or months.

In addition to the gate mechanism at spinal cord level, a pain inhibiting system also comes into play. This mechanism probably explains acupuncture's long-term pain relief. Greater weight is accorded nowadays to this pain inhibiting system, which allows for, among other things, a release of serotonin and noradrenaline (a hormone which is also a transmitter substance). At spinal cord level there are also receptors that work with dynorphin (one of the most efficient pain-relieving endorphins).

What happens in the central nervous system

The reticular system (RS, substantia reticularis) is thought to play a central role in ear acupuncture. This is a network of nerve fibres which connects the spinal cord with the brainstem, the hypothalamus area, the midbrain and the cortex. Through stimulating the reticular system one can influence muscle tone, breathing, blood pressure, electroencephalogram (EEG) and wakefulness. The RS can reduce, inhibit or strengthen both sensory and motor impulses. Like other reflex theories, ear acupuncture uses the reticular system as a pathway (Coutté & Zorn 1999).

---

[12] Substance P is a transmitter substance for pain, among other things.

[13] Bradykinin is an amino acid which, among other things, influences muscle contraction and the experiencing of pain.

[14] A growth hormone release inhibiting hormone.

[15] Vasoactive intestinal peptide, a tissue hormone which, among other things, widens the arteries and can inhibit the secretion of hydrochloric acid in the stomach.

Through upward-leading pathways acupuncture reaches the brainstem (nucleus raphee magnus locus ceruleus), PAG (periaquaductal grey) and thereafter the hypothalamus[16] and the thalamus[17] in the diencephalon.[18]

During acupuncture specific nuclei in the thalamus are activated. So too are unspecified nuclei which inhibit the feelings of discomfort generated by pain. At the same time there is less activity in the S2 area of the cortex (where the impression of pain is strengthened). On their way to the thalamus, signals are sent from the pathways to other parts of the brain. The effect of acupuncture is a result of collaboration between several centres of the brain.

Acupuncture results in the dampening of pain impulses not just in the central nervous system but also in the peripheral nervous system via signals transmitted from the central nervous system. It starts in the nucleus raphée magnus and is transmitted by, primarily, serotonin. Other substances such as endorphins and non-opioid substances such as noradrenaline, substance P and GABA are also involved in the dampening of pain impulses. Acupuncture achieves a change in the autonomic system, a sympathetic blockade, via a rearrangement in the hypothalamus.

Neurotransmitters and hormones

In the nervous system substances are produced which connect nerve impulses between the different cells and parts of the brain. These substances are released from nerve ends, circulate in the blood and activate or inhibit the functioning of organs. New substances are constantly being discovered. Amongst the better known are endorphins, serotonin, insulin,[19] adrenaline,[20] noradrenaline, acetylcholine,[21] dopamine,[22] histamine[23] and various hormones. The hormones guide and are in turn guided by the functioning of the hormonal glands (the pituitary, thyroid, parathyroid, pancreas, the ovaries and testicles). The amounts of these substances decide how we feel, both physically and psychologically. Researchers have studied which neurotransmitters and hormones in the blood and cerebrospinal fluid are involved during acupuncture. A large number of around 90 known neurotransmitters and many of the hormones are affected.

Endorphins

The neurotransmitters that are most often talked about in connection with acupuncture are the endorphins. Several studies have shown that both ear acupuncture and body acupuncture raise the levels of beta-endorphins, enkephalins (a subfraction of

---

[16] The hypothalamus is the basal part of the midbrain, part of the limbic system, and contains, among other things, the pituitary. It is via the pituitary that the hypothalamus governs both the autonomous and hormonal system. The pituitary receives impulses from the hypothalamus and releases different hormones.

[17] The thalamus lies under the cortex of the brain. Impulses 'pass through' the thalamus on their way from the body to the cortex.

[18] The diencephalon is the middle part of the brain. In the midbrain thirst, hunger, body temperature, sleep, menstruation, breathing, feelings and aggressions are regulated.

[19] A hormone which is produced in the pancreas and which influences sugar levels.

[20] Adrenaline, produced in the adrenal gland, is a neurotransmitter in the sympathetic nervous system.

[21] Acetylcholine is a tissue hormone which, among other things, helps to lower blood pressure and dilate blood vessels.

[22] Dopamine is a neurotransmitter which is a precursor to adrenaline and noradrenaline.

[23] Histamine is a tissue hormone released mostly in cases of allergy.

endorphin which occurs where opiate receptors are to be found) and dynorphin (the endorphin with the greatest capacity for pain relief) in the blood and spinal fluid. According to earlier scientific studies, endorphins are released during bodily exertion, massage, painful stimulation, stress and acupuncture. Endorphins are of great importance in pain relief and exert considerable influence over how we feel mentally.

Morphine-like substances such as alpha- and beta-endorphins are released partly where the needle penetrates the skin, partly in the central nervous system. Enkephalins (leu-enkephalin and met-enkephalin) are responsible for presynaptic inhibition of pain (they stop the pain impulses from reaching the cortex and the consciousness). During treatment of pain with acupuncture it is these mechanisms, among others, that come into effect.

More modern research has called into question the older theories concerning the increase in endorphins both during acupuncture and exercise. This shows that both endorphins and ACTH (which affects the level of cortisol) are stress hormones released during painful stimulation. Acupuncture with painfully high stimulation of the needles and physical strain which goes far beyond normal exercise should then trigger a heightening of endorphin levels. During more careful forms of acupuncture and in normal exercise such as jogging, according to these newer theories other mechanisms than the release of endorphins come into play, giving the pleasant relaxed feeling that many experience after acupuncture treatment and physical exercise.

Endorphins do not just influence the way we experience pain. They are thought to also have a direct influence on the appetite and on all forms of addiction. Earlier research ascribed a great part of the effect of acupuncture to endorphins. Now we know that many more mechanisms are involved. In treatment of withdrawal and the craving for drugs, part of the effect of treatment is related to the release of endorphins.

Endorphins bond easily with the body's receptors. This bonding occurs primarily during the first two weeks of withdrawal. That's why it is important that there should be frequent treatment during the first weeks. This response is the same, be it alcohol, medicinal or narcotic abuse.

It is interesting to note that levels of methionine in the brain, which are heightened in schizophrenic patients, are influenced by acupuncture (Karavis 1997).

Oxytocin

Oxytocin has received a great deal of attention in recent years. It lessens anxiety and is known as 'the feel-good hormone'. It appears to have a positive long term effect on conditions involving stress. Oxytocin levels are not only heightened during acupuncture but also when we laugh, touch and are touched, or undergo heat treatment or massage.

In order to maximise the calming effect of acupuncture, the therapist should increase conditions for high oxytocin levels by touching the patient, placing a warm rice pillow over the shoulders and giving non-painful acupuncture.

Placebo mechanisms

Just like all other treatments, acupuncture has its placebo effect. During medicinal treatment, the placebo effect can be so powerful that a patient may experience serious side effects from 'sugar pills' if they believe that they contain an active substance with which they cannot cope. The types of treatment that usually have a greater placebo effect are those which involve personnel in talking to or touching the patient. Invasive treatments, those involving a penetration of the skin, give rise to the greatest placebo effect. Surgery is an invasive treatment, as is acupuncture. Thus such treatments can have a greater placebo effect than, for example, medicines. In addition, the acupuncturist has the opportunity to touch and talk to the patient in peace and quiet. Ear acupuncture invites conversation without confrontation. If treatment can be given in such a way that the patient feels secure and well looked after, beneficial effects will be optimised.

The effect of acupuncture, and of ear acupuncture, is far greater than placebo. But the placebo effect is a bonus. We should be happy about this and take account of it when we administer acupuncture — precisely as in surgery, medication and other forms of treatment.

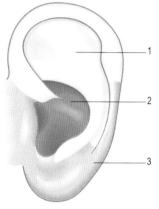

Figure 5.1 The ear is mainly innervated by three nerves:

1. Trigeminal nerve
2. Vagus nerve
3. Plexus cervicalis

Anatomy and innervation of the ear

When one explains from a Western perspective how acupuncture works, it becomes interesting to look in more detail at the nerves which serve the ear. The ear is richly innervated. At least three nerves serve the external ear: the trigeminal nerve, the great auricular nerve (nervus auricularis magnus) and the vagus nerve (see Fig. 5.1). The vagus nerve is perhaps the most interesting from our point of view.

Located on the surface of the ear, between epidermis and subcutis, there are around 10 000 sensory receptors which make it possible for the ear to be used in diagnosis and treatment. The ear also has a network of arteries, veins and lymph vessels.

The vagus nerve innervates the skin in part of the ear. The ear is the only place on the body where this nerve, via an extension, goes right to the surface of the skin. The vagus nerve serves primarily the internal organs in the thorax and abdomen. By stimulating the extension of the vagus nerve in the ear, it is possible via that nerve to influence the functioning of the internal organs.

When the ear is stimulated, for example by an acupuncture needle, a pellet or by warmth, the stimuli are registered by sensory receptors in the skin of the ear. The impulse is conducted to the central nervous system, the brain. A stimulus in the right ear goes to the left half of the brain because the nerve pathways cross the midline of the brain. Damage to the right elbow for example will, for the same reason, be 'registered' in the left half of the brain. The damage can be 'monitored' and treated in the right ear, because both the information from the injured body part to the brain and from the brain to the reflex point in the ear cross the midline of the brain.

More on the anatomy of the ear will be found in Ch. 6, The ear: its parts and acupuncture points.

The human being as a computer

The following is an unscientific model of thinking which is often used in seeking to understand the relationship of the ear to the brain: picture the human being as a computer. The ear is both the screen where we can see the information stored in the computer, and the keyboard which makes it possible to influence and programme the brain's functions. Through the keyboard we make contact with the body's central microprocessor, the brain. We can lose or damage an ear without destroying the brain/computer, but in so doing we lose the possibility of reading on the screen — diagnosing — and programming — treating — via the ear.

Somatotopic map

An explanation as to how acupuncture works, which applies only to certain forms of the treatment (above all ear acupuncture, but also acupuncture practised on the scalp, ankles and wrists, plus Su Jok and some other systems) builds on the idea of a microsystem or a somatotopy (see Ch. 4, Other microsystems). In a microsystem the whole of the body is represented in one part of the body. Each body part and organ has a corresponding point in another part of the body, for example in the ear or on the sole of the foot. A systematic representation of the body exists too in the cortex of the brain. This brain map has the same all-embracing pattern as the somatotopy that Nogier discovered in the ear in the 1950s. He found a bodily reproduction, a map, in the ear which shows a human being turned upside down. It is this reproduction of the whole body in one of its parts that we use in ear acupuncture.

There is a connection between the point in the ear and the brain and between the brain and the body part to which the point corresponds. Impulses between the brain and the somatotopic maps, such as that in the ear, go in both directions.

More somatotopies are briefly described in Ch. 4, Other microsystems.

Embryological explanations

Ear acupuncture books sometimes refer to an embryological[24] hypothesis which seeks to explain how the ear's reflex map relates to the rest of the body. On the one hand, the embryological hypothesis is based on the development of the ear in the foetus and the adult ear's nerve network. On the other hand, it makes use of a general anatomical knowledge of the way in which organs and tissues develop from the foetus's three germ layers, the endoderm, ectoderm and mesoderm.[25] The germ layers become specialised into different types of organs so that each one of these types of tissue is responsible for one of the human being's three systems of organs.

The ear is one of the few anatomic structures which are built up of tissue from each of these three primary tissue types to be found in an embryo. Paul Nogier maintained that each tissue type in the ear had a link to the various somatotopical reflections and to the innervation related to that part of the ear. The ear is innervated to a large degree by three nerves (see figure on page 49). In the zones innervated by each of these nerves there are differing distances between the receptors, as is the case concerning the different parts of the body innervated by these nerves. The more primitive internal organs have the least number of receptors. There are several receptors in the more developed muscular-skeletal tissue and most in the central nervous system.

---

[24] Embryology is the science of the foetus's development. The embryological hypothesis of ear acupuncture was launched in the 1970s by — among others — Bourdiol of France, and has since then received the support of other researchers, for example Durinjan in Russia.

[25] When an egg cell and sperm are united, rapid cell division starts. The first clump of cells is divided up into three different types, the endoderm, ectoderm and mesoderm.

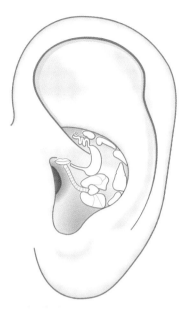

Figure 5.2 Internal organs originating in the endoderm are represented in the part of the ear innervated by the vagus nerve.

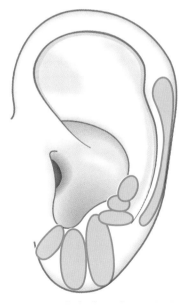

Figure 5.3 Body parts with an origin in the ectoderm are to be found represented in the part of the ear innervated by plexus cervicalis.

Endoderm

The endoderm gives rise to most of the internal organs (except for the heart and the kidneys): the stomach and intestinal system, lungs, tonsils, liver, pancreas, bladder, urinary system, thyroid, parathyroid and thymus. The organs are represented in the concha, the part of the ear served by the vagus nerve (see Fig. 5.2).

Ectoderm

The ectoderm gives rise to the skin, the brain, the spinal cord, subcortex, cortex and peripheral nerves, pineal gland, pituitary gland, kidney marrow, hair, nails, sweat glands, cornea, teeth, the mucous membrane of the nose, and the lenses of the eye (see Fig. 5.3). The part of the ear where these organs are found represented is served by a branch of plexus cervicalis which has indirect connections with the cortex. In the ear the organs are represented in the lobe and the tail of the helix.

Mesoderm

The mesoderm gives rise to the skeletal muscles, smooth muscle, blood vessels, bone, cartilage, joints, connective tissue, endocrine glands, kidney cortex, heart muscle, urogenital organ, uterus, fallopian tube, testicles and blood cells from the spinal cord and lymphatic tissue (see Fig. 5.4). The part of the ear where these organs are represented is served by the trigeminal nerve which supplies the brainstem with pain-blocking impulses for the muscles and skeleton. The organs are to be found represented in the antihelix, the scapha and fossa triangularis.

Laterality

Some researchers, Paul and Raphael Nogier among them, say that during treatment with ear acupuncture one should take account of laterality, the asymmetrical functioning of the two halves of the brain. Laterality influences the choice of acupuncture points and, above all, which ear should be treated.

Laterality refers to the way in which the halves of the brain cooperate. The right half of the brain controls the left side of the body and vice versa. The right and left halves of the brain have different, specific functions. Both are important.

How the two halves of the brain cooperate

A human being's personality and condition depends in part on how the halves of the brain cooperate. The left half is used to learn languages, how to write, count and read, to think logically and solve problems rationally. The right half is important for understanding and describing music, colours, form and rhythm and for creativity, intuition and spontaneity. Artists are more often left-handed than scientists and vice versa.

The two halves of the brain are attached by the corpus callosum. This consists of 20 million nerve fibres and forms a 'bridge' between the two halves of the brain. If the 'passage is free' impulses can connect between the two halves, something which is of importance, for example, when it comes to simultaneous capacity, the ability to do two things at the same time. Communication between the two halves of the brain is decisive in determining how a person functions. If communication is broken, the two halves work on their own, which makes it difficult for a person to have an all-round perspective. If the passage in the corpus callosum is completely broken off (due to an operation, for example), the two halves each work on their own, without the right hand knowing what the left hand is doing, and vice versa. Contact between the two halves of the brain is considered to be favourably influenced by exercises in which the body moves diagonally (movements where the right hand meets the left foot and vice versa, such as crawling, rolling and cross-country skiing).

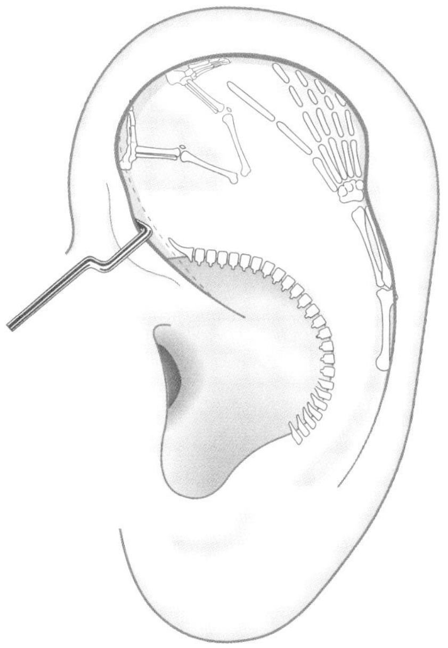

Humanity has a dominant side

No other species apart from human beings are either right- or left-handed. Even chimpanzees, which most resemble humans, use either their right or left hands and feet with no apparent difficulty.[26] On the other hand, even when newborn, human babies show a tendency towards one side or the other. The child develops in phases in which the dominance of one side or the other becomes more or less apparent. Around six years of age the child is permanently either left or right handed. Ninety-eight percent of adults are right-handed (and thus possess a dominant left half of the brain), while just 2 percent are left-handed (Coutté & Zorn 1999).

Human beings thus have a dominant half, which Nogier calls a laterality. If the left half of the brain is dominant, you'll be right-handed and if the right half is dominant then you'll be left-handed. If a right-handed person is able to use his right hand and a left-handed person is able to and allowed to use his left hand, there are no problems. But if you are not allowed to use your dominant hand but are forced to use the 'wrong' hand, then a laterality disturbance may occur. In times gone by it was common for people born left-handed to be forced or 'taught' to use their right hand instead.[27] When a person is not sure which side is the dominant one, or the communication between the two halves of the brain functions badly, a pathology may occur (Coutté & Zorn 1999). A laterality disturbance can be generated by injury and can give rise to malfunctioning. Laterality problems are often cited in connection with dyslexia, stammering, bedwetting and difficulties in learning.

Figure 5.4 Body parts with an origin in the mesoderm are represented in the part of the ear served by the trigeminal nerve.

---

[26] In 2003 *BMC Ecology* published an article about walruses on Greenland. For the first time researchers were able to show that a creature living in water was right 'flippered'. The walrus had, according to the article, more powerful frontal thrust on the right side and dug after eating mostly with the right flipper.
[27] According to Nogier the reverse can also happen if a right-handed person works a great deal with the right half of the brain, for example in expressing artistic form. Nogier said that people with certain professions belong to a risk group for laterality disturbance. In particular actors but also artists, musicians and dancers use one side of their brain more than the other.

It is not possible to train away left-handedness. If a left-handed child is compelled to use the right hand then it learns to use the emotional half of the brain for logical thinking. This can, according to Raphael Nogier, create a personality that is impulsive, emotional and irrational. A boy (90 percent of such cases are boys) can begin to stammer (the speech centre is in the left half of the brain) and have difficulties in school with spelling and concentration. As an adult he may suffer from several psychosomatic problems. He can have problems both at work and in relationships because he uses the emotional half of the brain to deal with technical questions and applies the logical half to human relations.

Temporary disturbances in laterality

Nogier said that laterality problems can occur in people whose brain halves previously worked well together, in cases when one loses balance, laterality, in existence. Contributory factors can be physical, such as concussion, or psychological trauma like stress, sorrow, lack of sleep or shock. Neuroleptica, withdrawal from tobacco (Coutté & Zorn 1999), systemic diseases and neurological diseases such as multiple sclerosis (MS) can, according to Nogier, cause laterality disturbance. Many of us have, at some period of our life, suffered from temporary laterality imbalance.

Treating the dominant ear

In ear acupuncture treatment is normally given to the ear which is on the same side as the part of the body causing pain. If there is pain in the right knee then as a rule, the right ear should be treated. If the treatment is given for a condition which is not situated either to right or left, for example constipation or allergy, then usually the dominant ear is treated (the right ear for right-handed patients and the left for left-handed patients).

If a patient has a laterality problem, Nogier says it is important to treat it before other problems are dealt with (see Ch. 11, Method and Ch. 12, Treatment suggestions). Finding out which side is dominant is called laterality testing. For methods of testing laterality, see Ch. 10, Examination of the ear.

The ear: its parts and acupuncture points

Chapter contents

What exactly is an ear?

'Ear is an organ of hearing symmetrically on both sides of the head', it says in one textbook (Xinnong 1987). Another states: 'The auricle is an oval elastic structure of subtemporal position between the mandibular joint and the mastoid. At its vertical longitudinal axis, this oval structure measures approximately 60–65 mm, while the horizontal diameter is approximately 30–35 mm' (Rubach 2001). In medical terminology 'ear' is defined as 'a paired organ for hearing and balance'. The inner ear, which cannot be seen in a general inspection from the outside, contains the building blocks that allow us to hear (see Fig. 6.1). The external ear, on the other hand, has very little to do with hearing. While the external ear acts as a funnel, catching and amplifying sound waves and thus contributing to better hearing, a person without an external ear can still have good hearing.

However, let's be thankful that we do have an external ear. It's actually a tremendously practical piece of anatomy. In part it provides us with a wonderful reflex map of the rest of the body so that we can quite easily investigate bodily disorders. In addition, we can use the same organ to treat any imbalance that we find.

The ear is constructed at an early stage during the development of the foetus in the uterus. When it is 25 days old, the two large cavities that are the beginnings of the ear can be seen quite clearly. Before the external ear is created, the middle and inner ears are formed, making it possible for the baby to hear and to have a properly functioning sense of balance. By the 12th week of pregnancy the external ear is clearly

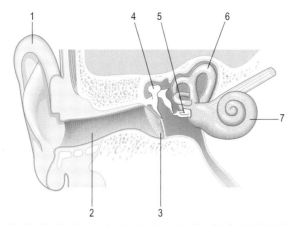

Figure 6.1 The inner ear.

1. The external ear
2. External ear canal
3. Eardrum, or tympanum
4. Hammer, or malleus
5. Stirrup
6. Semicircular canals
7. Cochlea

visible and six weeks later the ear is complete and the foetus can, during the last five months in the uterus, hear (Nilsson & Hemberger 2004).

The middle ear consists of the eardrum and the three hearing bones (or ossicles, namely the malleus or hammer, the incus or anvil and the stapes or stirrup), the Eustachian tube and tympanic cavity. The inner ear consists of the labyrinth containing the hearing organs, the cochlea and semicircular canals, which help us to balance.

The external ear comprises a plate of elastic cartilage, forming a complex pattern, and a layer of fat and tissue. All is covered with skin and served by different nerves, blood and lymph vessels. The upper portion of the ear contains more cartilage, while the lobe consists mostly of soft tissue.

Skin

The skin consists of several layers of cells and has many more functions than that of just being a 'bag' containing the other organs. Via the skin we regulate, among other things, warmth and disposal of waste products. The skin also has a complex bioelectromagnetic activity.

Sensory receptors

To understand more easily how the ear can be used for diagnosis and treatment consider the fact that in the borderland between the outer, leathery layer of skin, the epidermis, and the second and third layers, the dermis and hypodermis, there are around 10 000 special sensory receptors, at most 0.1 mm large. They are made up of collagen fibres and are surrounded by a membrane containing a negative electrical charge. Each point in the ear contains a group of these sensors (five per square millimetre), which are served by the same nerve and vessel stem. Among other things the receptors react to mechanical pressure (such as pressure from a pressure pen or pricking with a needle), heat (for example from moxibustion[1] or burning with a piece of hot metal) and stimuli such as laser light and electrical stimulation. The receptors forward the information to the brain.

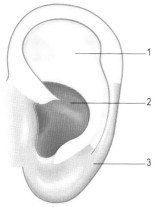

Figure 6.2 The ear is served in the main by three nerves:

1. Trigeminal nerve
2. Vagus nerve
3. Plexus cervicalis

Nerves

When we try to explain how ear acupuncture works from a Western viewpoint, it becomes interesting to study the nerves that serve the ear (see Fig. 6.2). Several different nerves[2] are involved. The sensors are innervated by three types of nerve fibres. These are sensory nerves, sympathetic and parasympathetic nerve fibres from the vagus nerve and the glossopharyngeal nerve. The border between the fields of the various nerves is not clearly defined, they overlap one another.

In this connection, the vagus nerve is perhaps the most interesting. The vagus is the tenth cranial nerve, a mixed nerve with a large area to cover. It is both a sensory and a motor nerve and has connections with the parasympathetic nerve fibres to the internal organs in the abdomen and thorax. The vagus nerve innervates the skin of just one body part, the concha of the ear. There the vagus nerve penetrates the elastic cartilage in the ear and spreads out over the surface of the concha and round the external ear canal. It is in just this area that most internal organs are represented by their reflex points. This may explain how by stimulating zones in the ear one can influence internal organs and that the internal organ can 'leave a message' which can be read by the skin.[3]

Why some people cough, yawn or feel ill when they poke around in the ear may be explained as an stimulation of the vagus nerve.

Blood vessels

In the ear there is a network of arteries,[4] which provides the tissue with fresh oxygen, and veins,[5] which transport the blood back to the heart. The blood vessels in the ear are small. In the lobe are slightly larger vessels which make it possible to take samples of capillary blood from the earlobe. In ear acupuncture it is unusual for bleeding to occur. When the needle is removed there can sometimes come one

---

[1] Treatment with moxa, a herb the Chinese have used for thousands of years to warm points on the skin. See Ch. 2, A brief look at traditional Chinese medicine (TCM).

[2] Among them the facial nerve (the seventh cranial nerve which serves the ear's rudimentary muscles in the concha and in certain individual places on and behind the ear), the vagus nerve, the trigeminal nerve (fifth cranial nerve), glossopharyngealis, cervical plexus and the great auricular nerve, nervus auriculus magnus.

[3] Carlsson (1992) writes: 'Thus it is in the area innervated by the vagus that reflex points for all the inner organs are situated. Other areas are principally innervated by the trigeminal and great auricular nerve (C2-3). So there are anatomical conditions for different interreactions at a high cervical level (the trigeminal reaches here) and also conditions for changeovers in the vagus nerve'.

[4] Among them arteria temporalis superficialis to the front of the ear and arteria auricularis posterior on its rear.

[5] Among them vena jugularis interna to the back and front of the ear.

or two drops of blood. Such bleeding is easily stopped by pressing a cotton bud to the point for a few seconds.

Lymph vessels

The external ear is covered with a network of lymph vessels. Their job is to drain unwanted substances.

What is an ear acupuncture point?

If some part of the body experiences pain, stress, malfunctioning or illness, a reflex point will be created at the corresponding area in the ear. The area often becomes very sore. Sometimes a change may be seen with the naked eye, sometimes it feels as if there is a small grain of sand under the skin in the affected area. The electrical resistance of the skin is changed so that the point can also be found with an electrical point detector. An active point can also be warmer or colder than the surrounding tissue and can therefore also be found with an instrument for measuring temperature.[6]

The definition of an active ear acupuncture point is a point in the ear that becomes sore if pressed and/or has changed skin resistance if tested with an electrical instrument and/or has changed colour, or can be felt as a tiny bump about the size of a grain of sand, or as a cavity. An active point is also called a painful, sensitive, irritated or reaction point. The most common method of finding active points is to look for them with a probe or with an electrical point detector.

How many points are there in the ear?

The 365 acupuncture points on the body may always be found with an electrical point detector.[7] This contrasts with the ear where points are active only if there is something wrong with the corresponding body part. The points in the ear are part of a reflex system and are either 'on' or 'off'. They can be found only when there is a disturbance in the corresponding organ. When tested with a probe or with an electrical point detector, a person who is 100 percent healthy should therefore show no points. Some points in the ear are an exception to this rule, however. On most people an electrical point detector will find Point Zero, Shen Men or some of the other so-called masterpoints.

On a totally healthy person the point corresponding to the stomach can become active after a large meal because then the stomach may be overloaded. Similarly, the Endocrine point becomes active in healthy women during menstruation, if they are in puberty or menopause, not because they are sick but because their hormone levels are unstable. In other words, not all active points need to be treated.

If you look at an ear acupuncture point map, you will find up to 200 points noted. Several of them are — more accurately — zones. The map should be seen only as a guide. If an organ is overloaded or sick an active point may be found in the zone but it can move a little from day to day. Therefore it is important on each

---

[6] Marignan conducted research into this in the 1990s. The measuring of points by temperature is a method that has been developed no further and is not normally used in the clinical world.

[7] Body points are 'openings' on the meridians, the channels in which energy constantly flows, see Ch. 2, A brief look at traditional Chinese medicine (TCM).

occasion to search for active points in order to be able to pierce them as accurately as possible.

In Ch. 10, Examination of the ear, I describe how to look for the active points and in Ch. 11, Method, how they should be treated.

The topography of the ear

Ears can be very different from one another. One person may have flat ears with tough cartilage, another ears with a soft layer of tissue over the cartilage. A third may have ears that are a richly sculptured, three dimensional work of art, with deep creases and clear structure. Ears can be small or large, elongated or rounded. In the examples below, an average ear is described. You will see many variations from the norm. If uncertain as to what's what when examining an ear, you can always be sure the active points you find are worth treating.

Terminology

In order to understand and describe where a point is located, it is a good idea to know the names of the various parts of the ear. I use Latin names such as helix, scaphoid fossa and tragus but for other points use the colloquial English version. For example the 'antihelix crus inferior' is referred to as 'the lower leg of the antihelix'.

The names of the points

Each point has, since the beginnings of ear acupuncture, been given various names because different authors and translators have chosen different terminology in the books that have been published on the method. Sometimes the point will have been named after the organ for which it is a reflex point, for example Liver or Shoulder. In other cases the points bear the names of the condition to be treated, for example Aggression or Constipation. Certain authors have chosen to name the points after medicines which have a similar effect, for example the Valium point or the Barbiturate Analogue point. Some points have been named after a person, for example Jerome's point and the R-point (after Roger Bourdiol).

To avoid misunderstanding in the text I have chosen to spell the name of the point with an initial capital. The point corresponding to the knee is thus written Knee.

The points which are noted differently on French or Chinese maps have F (French point) or C (Chinese point) in parenthesis after the name. For example: Kidney (C), Kidney (F).

In some cases I have chosen to use the generally accepted Chinese terminology. For example: Shen Men (Spirit Gate or Divine Gate), San Jiao (Triple Heater, Triple Energizer).

From points to zones

Certain parts of the ear have a good many points with a similar function described in different books. In some places I have chosen to bring together these points to a zone and to give it a single name. In acupuncture literature you can find, for example, on the inside of the antitragus points with names such as Thalamus, Subcortex, Middle Border, Nervus,

Pain Control Point and Dermis. I have chosen to describe them as a point/zone with the name Thalamus.

Towards the front of the lobe there are points with names such as Master Omega, Master Cerebral, Omega O, Nervosity, Neurasthenia, Anxiety point, Psychosomatic and the Bromazepam Analogue Point. These points I have chosen to describe as a zone which I call Master Cerebral.

Another example is the hormonal zone. In this zone are points with names such as FSH (Follicle Stimulating Hormone), LH (Luteinizing Hormone), ACTH (Adrenocorticotrophic Hormone), TSH (Thyroid Stimulating Hormone), Gonadotrophin, Oxytocin and Vasopressin. I have chosen to call the zone containing all these points Endocrine.

Positions

In medical terminology, when describing where parts of the body are located in relation to one another, Latin terms are used, such as medial (close to the body's middle line), lateral (away from the body's middle line), distal (away from the centre of the body) and proximal (closer to the centre of the body). To simplify matters I have chosen another way to describe the relationship of the points to one another. This takes as its starting point a patient in a sitting position and gives the position of the points in the ear according to the following principles:

'In front' = closer to the patient's nose.
Example: 'Large Intestine lies in front of Small Intestine.'
'Behind' = closer to the patient's neck.
Example: 'Bladder lies behind Urethra.'
'Above' = closer to the crown of the patient's head.
Example: 'Shen Men lies above Kidney.'
'Below' = further away from the crown of the patient's head.
Example: 'Shoulder lies below Elbow.'

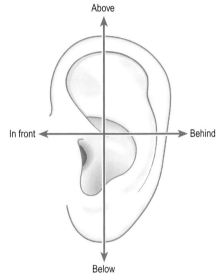

Figure 6.3 Description of the position of points.

Landmarks of the ear

Ears can look very different from one another. In order to describe the placement of a certain point, specific orienteering points, or landmarks are used. These pinpoint the area containing the point or zone you are looking for. Oleson (2003) uses a system of 18 landmarks (LM), numbered from LM 0 to LM 17 (see Fig. 6.4). Twelve of them will be used as reference points in this book. They have been given the same numbering that Oleson used.

Parts of the ear

The ear's various parts and their names are listed below. Acupuncture points in the ear are divided up according to a special pattern. There follows a broad outline of which reflex points are to be found in the various parts of the ear.

An upside down human being is reflected in the ear. One of the most popular representations of this is a picture of a little child huddled up in the foetal position in the form of the external ear. A more correct

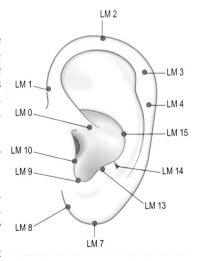

Figure 6.4 Landmarks (LM) referred to in the text.

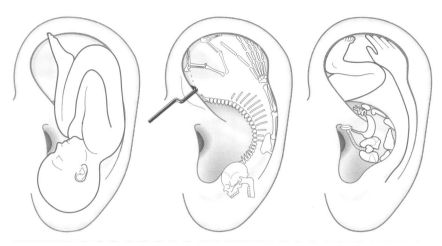

Figure 6.5 An upside-down human being is reflected in the ear. In the ear to the left we see the picture of the little child, huddled together in the foetal position and with a form that resembles the external ear. The other two pictures show more accurately how the reflex points are divided up in the ear. The reflected human being stands on his head with the skull and face reflected in the lobe, the internal organs in the concha, the backbone along the antihelix, the arm in the scaphoid fossa and the leg in the fossa triangularis and at the upper leg of the antihelix.

representation of how the reflex points are divided up in the ear shows a more twisted human being. It is standing on its head, with the skull and face represented in the lobe, the internal organs in the concha, the backbone along the antihelix, the arm in the scaphoid fossa, and the leg in the fossa triangularis and in the upper leg of the antihelix (see Figs 6.5 and 6.6).

The upper root of the ear

The upper root of the ear is its highest point, where it is joined to the head. The upper root is LM 1, (landmark 1, see Fig. 6.4).

The lower root of the ear

Similarly, the lower root of the ear is the lowest point where it is joined to the head. The lower root is LM 8. If a person has a small ear lobe, LM 8 can be located below LM 7.

Helix

Helix is Latin for spiral. It is the name given for the edge of the ear. The helix begins in the middle of the ear as a raised ridge known as the helix root. The helix root usually runs horizontally along the bottom of the concha. Sometimes the helix root will end sloping backwards/downwards. The helix root can seldom be discerned in the rear portion of the concha but in the middle of the concha it appears as a clearly formed ridge. In the front part there is a vertical notch over the helix root. It can be felt if you draw a fingernail or a screwdriver-like object along the helix root. In this notch can be found the landmark point LM 0, which is also Point Zero (see Ch. 8, Functional points.)

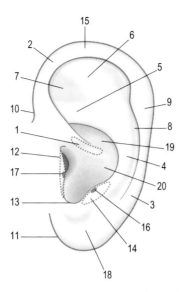

Figure 6.6 Parts of the ear.

1. Helix root
2. The ascending part of helix
3. The helix tail
4. Antihelix
5. Antihelix — lower leg
6. Antihelix — upper leg
7. Fossa triangularis
8. Scaphoid fossa
9. Darwin's tubercle
10. The ear's upper root
11. The ear's lower root
12. Tragus
13. Incisura intertragica
14. Antitragus
15. Apex
16. Antitragus apex
17. Tragus apex
18. The ear lobe
19. Cymba concha, upper part of concha
20. Cavum concha, lower part of concha

Behind Point Zero on the helix root lies the Stomach point and in front of it points that correspond to the genitalia.

The ascending part of helix then runs forward and upwards round the ear. On most ears the edge of the helix is folded inwards towards the centre of the ear. Sometimes it is so tightly folded that you cannot see the inside of the helix without opening the edge and bending it out. In other ears there is only the hint of a fold.

On the upper part of the descending helix a visible thickening of the helix occurs. This is known as Darwin's tubercle and is a leftover from mankind's evolution. On animals Darwin's tubercle forms the top of the ear. Directly across the helix above and below Darwin's tubercle there is often a little notch which can be felt if you draw a fingernail across the helix. This forms landmarks (LM) 3 and 4.

The helix then disappears into the ear lobe. The lowest part of the helix is referred to as its tail.

On the helix can be found, among other points, several tonsil points. On the edge of the helix are also several landmarks (LM). The ear's topmost point, the apex, forms LM 2. The lowest part of the lobe is LM 7. LM 3 lies at the upper border of Darwin's tubercle and LM 4 on the lower border.

Apex

The highest point of the ear is called the apex and is LM 2. The apex is a part of the helix. On, or close to the apex, you'll find the functional point Allergy. (The tips of the tragus and the antihelix are also referred to as 'apexes'.)

Antihelix

The antihelix is the raised, thick ridge which runs upwards parallel with the helix in the centre of the ear. It bends forward and divides into two legs. The lower leg (crus inferior) is slender and protruding, the upper leg (crus superior) is wider and often flatter.

Along the forward edge, the wall, of the ascending antihelix and the edge below the lower leg of the antihelix which together frame the concha, are several parallel zones. Closest to the edge can be found a zone with the points representing the vertebrae of the backbone. Next to and below that zone, closer to the concha, runs a parallel zone. Here the discs are represented. Next to that zone, even closer to the concha, is a third zone with points which, via the nervous system, influence the hormonal glands: thyroid, parathyroid, thymus, pancreas, the mammary glands and the adrenal glands.

In front of/below this zone there is another zone which represents the sympathetic trunk (a nerve running parallel with the backbone on the outside of the vertebrae. The sympathetic trunk plays a significant role in the functioning of the internal organs in the thorax and abdomen) (see Fig. 6.7).

There are two landmarks on the antihelix. The crossing point between the antitragus and antihelix acts as a landmark, LM 14. LM 15 lies in a small groove on the antihelix where an extension of the helix root should have crossed the antihelix. Between LM 14 and LM 15 you'll find the reflex points for the cervical vertebrae.

According to the Chinese point map the leg and the foot are represented on the upper leg of the antihelix (crus superior).

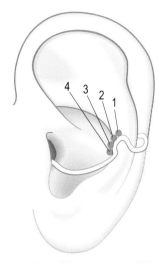

Figure 6.7 Four parallel zones along antihelix.

1. Reflex zone for the vertebrae
2. Reflex zone for the discs
3. Zone for the endocrine glands
4. Zone for the sympathetic trunk.

Fossa triangularis

Between the upper and lower legs of the antihelix there is a large depression. With a bit of imagination one can see it as a three-sided structure. For this reason it is known by the Latin term, fossa triangularis.

If you search for a point in the fossa triangularis and have difficulty making out its edges, try carefully pressing together the ear by pushing the upper and lower antihelix 'legs' against one another so that the cavity becomes visible. Look too at the colour and structure of the skin. Often the skin is darker and less shiny in the cavity which makes it easier to see where the cavity begins and ends.

According to the French point map, the leg and foot are represented in fossa triangularis. Here too lies one of the most frequently used ear acupuncture points, Shen Men.

Scapha, the scaphoid fossa

Scapha comes from the Greek *scaphos*, meaning 'small boat'. It is the depressed surface between the helix and antihelix. It is wider at the top and narrower at the bottom, like the blade of an oar, though the scaphoid fossa is seldom as straight as an oar but bowed with the oar blade facing forward.

In the scaphoid fossa you will find reflex points for Shoulder, Arm and Hand.

In its rear portion, concealed uder the edge of the helix, lies an oblong zone known as the vegetative groove. In this are reflex points used primarily in geometrical ear acupuncture for treatment of pain in the locomotor system. (See *Point Zero geometry*, page 171.)

Tragus and subtragus

The tragus is the piece of cartilage in front of the ear. Sometimes it is arched in the form of a bow, sometimes it consists of two bows. The top of the tragus is called the apex, as is the highest point of the ear. If the tragus has two bows it is the top of the lower bow which is the apex. The tragus apex is a landmark, LM 10. The inside of the tragus is called the subtragus.

On the tragus and subtragus are points which have an effect on the nose and ear, the adrenal gland, stress hormones, laterality, addiction etc.

Antitragus

The antitragus is the arch-shaped cartilage structure situated opposite and behind the tragus. One end of the antitragus starts at the incisura intertragica, which separates the tragus from the antitragus. The other end of the antitragus is connected with the antihelix. At this junction there is a notch which can be felt if you draw a fingernail or a screwdriver-like tool along the edge. The notch corresponds to the point where the base of the skull joins the first cervical vertebra and is a landmark, LM 14.

The apex is the most distinctive part of the antitragus and is a landmark (LM 13). In the antitragus lie reflex points for parts of the cranium and brain.

Incisura intertragica

Incisura intertragica is Latin for 'the groove between the two traguses'. It is also sometimes called the intertragic notch. It is in this area that the Hormonal zone is to be found. Incisura intertragica is a landmark, LM 9.

The earlobe

The lobe is the soft part of the bottom part of the ear. Here there is no cartilage. The lobe can be divided into nine squares via a horizontal line drawn from the lower edge of the incisura intertragica (LM 9). Then two other horizontal lines are drawn to divide the lobe into three equal parts. These lines are bisected with two vertical lines to form three equal parts. The squares that are formed are then numbered from front to back, up and down, the square furthest to the front is number 1, that at the back of the bottommost line number 9. This makes it easier to describe the position of the points (see Fig. 6.8).

The lowest point of the ear lobe is a landmark, LM7.

In the middle of the lobe, in square number 5, is the Eye point. In the rest of the lobe are most of the other points representing the parts of the face and skull.

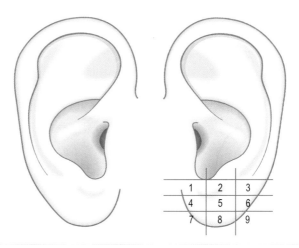

Figure 6.8 The earlobe is divided into nine squares.

The concha

The concha is a large cavity in the centre of the ear. It is surrounded by the tragus, the antitragus, the ascending part of the antihelix and the lower leg of the antihelix. The concha is divided into two parts. The upper part is called cymba[8] concha and the lower part the cavum[9] concha.

The external ear canal opens into the forward, upper corner of the cavum concha.

The internal organs are represented in the concha. In the upper part (above the helix root) are the intestines and the urinary system. In the lower part (below the helix root) is the mouth, oesophagus and respiratory organs.

The back of the ear

On the back of the ear are several of the frontal parts, only in negative relief — the concha, which turns inward on the front of the ear, bulges out on the backside, and the antihelix, which bulges out on the front of the ear, is a cavity on the backside (see Fig. 6.9).

Along the backside of the ear runs a vertical groove which corresponds to the antihelix on the opposite side. In the same way, as the antihelix divides into two 'legs' on the front of the ear, the furrow to the rear divides, to form a triangle. This furrow, with its backward extension, is often called the Blood Pressure Groove.

The part of the ear which lies between the groove and the skull is called the rear concha (Oleson 2003).

There is, of course, also a lobe on the rear of the ear.

On the back of the ear the same organs and parts of the body are represented as on the front. The points on the rear are thought above all to influence motor activity of the particular organ. In this book we shall look at only a few of the points on the back of the ear.

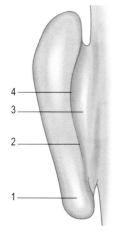

Figure 6.9 The back of the ear.

1. The back of the lobe
2. The back of the antihelix
3. The back of the concha
4. The Blood Pressure Groove

---

[8] Cymba is Latin for something resembling a boat.
[9] Cavum is Latin for emptiness, a vacant space, hollow, or a cave.

Reflex points and functional points

Broadly speaking, there are two types of points. The first are reflex points which correspond to parts of the body. They may also be called organ points. Every part of the body, whether a muscle, a bone, an internal organ or a blood vessel, has a reflex point in the ear. The reflex points are described in Ch. 7, Reflex points.

The second group are functional points. These are described in Ch. 8, Functional points. Unlike reflex points, functional points have what is known as a systemic effect. They influence not just a localised part of the body but have a general effect on bodily functions. The Allergy point is used, for example, as the name indicates, to diagnose and treat allergies and the Sympathetic Autonomic point has an effect on the autonomous nervous system. Other points have a recognisable effect on mental condition.

Many points, among them the points corresponding to parts of the brain, are at one and the same time both reflex and functional points. These points are discussed in Ch. 7, Reflex points. Some are also discussed in Ch. 8, Functional points.

Meridians in the ear?

According to TCM, meridians are channels where the qi, or life energy, flows (see Ch. 2, A brief look at traditional Chinese medicine). The Chinese think that in addition to all the various parts of the body, meridians are also represented in the ear. Nogier thought in a more Western way and said that meridians (which do not exist organically) were not represented in the ear.

If we take as our starting point the upside-down human being in the ear, some points are placed in unexpected places. The placing of many points is understandable if we think of the meridians and acupuncture points depicted on the upside-down figure in the ear. For example the Uterus (F) point in the fossa triangularis lies on the lower leg of the figure in the ear. On the actual lower leg there is an acupuncture point, SP6, which is one of the most important body acupuncture points when it comes to having an effect on the uterus.

Another example: The Insomnia 1 point lies in the scaphoid fossa, on the wrist of the figure in the ear. On the body's actual wrist there is a body acupuncture point, HT 7, which in body acupuncture is a cardinal point when treating insomnia (see Fig. 6.10).

The function of the points

We can't describe the effect of each and every one of the points with scientific exactitude, based on controlled, randomised, double-blind studies, because they have not been studied individually. In this book I base descriptions from the book *Chinese Acupuncture and Moxibustion* (Xinnong 1987), and works by Nogier (Coutté & Zorn 1988, 1999, Nogier & Nogier 1985), the research team of the Nanking Army Hospital (Huang 1974), Oleson (2003), Strittmatter (2003), Rubach (2001) and some other authors. I shall also use what I have been told by my own teachers of ear acupuncture[10] and draw on my own experience as an ear acupuncturist.

In the following chapters I shall describe where each point is located and the effect it is meant to have, according to those experts cited above. When Paul Nogier

---

[10] Among others Björn Överbye, Xiao Hui Shen, Raphael Nogier and Alain Coutté.

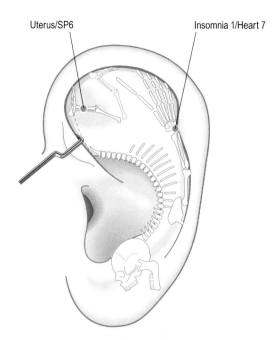

Uterus/SP6   Insomnia 1/Heart 7

Figure 6.10 Examples of how the functions of two points in the ear agree with the effect on two body acupuncture points, lying on a meridian running through the part of the body reflected in the same zones as the two ear acupuncture points.
1. The ear point Uterus (F) lies in the reflex zone for the lower leg. The spleen's meridian passes the lower leg and has its body acupuncture point SP 6 as a cardinal point used to treat gynaecological problems.
2. The ear point Insomnia 1 lies in the reflex zone for the wrist. The meridian for the heart passes through the body's wrist and on the heart meridian, close to the wrist is the point HT 7 used to treat disturbed sleep.

discovered the reflex points in the ear, he described them from a Western medical perspective. He did not consider qi, yin and yang or the meridians. The Chinese researchers who, around the same time as Nogier, presented their own version of the ear's reflex points, interpreted their discovery from the point of view of traditional Chinese medicine (TCM). They said the organ points were not just reflex points for individual organs but also could be used to treat other symptoms, which according to TCM are related to the organ in question. When it comes to certain points, I have included the effect described according to TCM. In such cases, I might say, for example: 'According to TCM the Hormonal point can also solve the problem of stagnated liver qi, activate the circulation of blood and lessen damp and oedema'. This is the sort of information that can be of use to people educated in TCM. Other readers can skip it. There is not space enough to go into the concepts on which TCM is based. Some of the books dealing with Chinese medicine are listed in the Bibliography at the end of this book. A short review of how TCM looks at the functioning of the human body and principles used in diagnosis and treatment can be found in Ch. 2, A brief look at traditional Chinese medicine (TCM).

Masterpoints

Masterpoints are points which have considerable effect. Some of them are active on most people. 'Primary masterpoints' is a concept that Oleson (1998) used for five points which give a particularly powerful effect. These are the Sympathetic Autonomic Point, Shen Men, Endocrine, Point Zero and Thalamus.

Oleson also named five 'secondary masterpoints', which are also unusually potent ear acupuncture points. These are: Allergy, Master Oscillation, Master Sensorial, Master Cerebral (the point sometimes called Master Omega) and the V-point. In the third edition of the same book Oleson (2003) abandons the concepts of 'primary' and 'secondary' and refers to all 10 points as simply 'masterpoints'. Masterpoints are described in Chapter 8, Functional points.

Giving priority to active points

It cannot be stressed enough that first and foremost it is active points that should be treated. Search for points that look different, are sore or have a changed skin resistance (See Ch. 10, Examination of the ear).

If no active points are found in the expected zones, one can still treat the zone where the point is meant to be according to the point map.

7

Reflex points

In this chapter we shall look at the points and zones in the ear that correspond to different parts of the body, the so-called reflex or organ points. First we'll look at the points which correspond to the locomotor system, then the reflex points for the head, the nervous system, sense organs and internal organs. Several points are both reflex and functional points, for example the points that represent the parts of the brain. You'll find some of them in both this chapter and Ch. 8, Functional points.

The points are named after the parts of the body they represent. In parentheses after the name of the points are alternative names given in different instruction books.

Those points, which are annotated differently on the French[1] and Chinese maps, have F (for French point) or C (Chinese point) in brackets after the name. Example: Kidney (F), Kidney (C).

Active points

Reflex points become active if the corresponding organ or body part is not functioning as it should. An active point can have changed colour, become sore, the skin can change structure and the bioelectrical activity can change so that you can find the point with an electrical point detector. (See Ch. 10, Examination of the ear.)

As a rule the reflex points become active in the ear on the same side of the body as the part where the pain is located. In the case of the right knee being injured, no matter whether the person is right- or left-handed, the Knee point will most often become active in the right ear. (However, functional points will as a rule become active either on both sides or on the dominant side, which is to say, on the right ear for a right-handed person and on the left for a left-handed person.)

---

[1] The first European point map was drawn up in France by Paul Nogier, who set the trend in ear acupuncture. Now other European researchers have published material on ear acupuncture. American authors have also named points. It would perhaps be more correct to label the non-Chinese points E for European or W for Western but for the sake of simplicity I have decided to keep to F for the non-Chinese points.

Understanding the illustrations

The 'open' ear: Used to show the location of the various ear acupuncture points. Those points that are hidden when looking straight at the ear are sometimes shown in an 'open' ear. In such illustrations the edges of the helix, tragus and antitragus are folded back and held in place with hooks so that the subtragus, the inside of the antitragus and the inside of the edge of the helix become visible. In reality, no hooks would be used, of course.

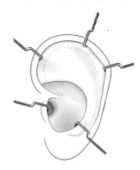

Different symbols are used to indicate the points:

● A bullet point means that the point is visible when viewed straight on.

▲ A triangle means that the point is concealed, for example, lies on the inside of the tragus, or behind the edge of the helix.

★ A star means that the point lies on the wall between the antihelix and the concha.

The placing of the points in the illustrations is schematic. Because no two ears are the same it is difficult to give an exact location. To actually locate active points in each individual ear, careful point finding is recommended.

How a reflex point is used in treatment

Every reflex point can be used to treat symptoms which the patient experiences in the corresponding part of the body. The Knee point is active and can be used to treat pain or injury to the patient's knee whether or not the wound is to a bone, tendon, ligament or muscle. In the same way, the Thumb point can be used for injury or pain in all parts of the thumb. The Thumb point becomes active if the thumb's skeletal structure, muscles, tendons or skin are injured. Even the blood vessels passing through the parts of the body are represented in the point.

Thus, muscular tension, weakness or trembling in a muscle, pain from a fracture, a swollen joint, or arthritic or rheumatic pain in a joint, skin irritation or even sunburn can be treated at the same point if the symptoms are in the same body part.

Difference in effect on points on the front and rear of the ear

The parts of the locomotor system are represented in one point on the front of the ear and another on the back. Most often they lie opposite one another. Often it is thought that the point on the front of the ear works best in the case of pain while the point to the rear is best treated for problems involving movement. Palpate both sides of the ear. If the patient experiences pain in — for example — a shoulder, you can treat the point on the front to relieve pain and the one to the rear to alleviate any muscular tension which can have developed as a result.

Balancing effect

Ear acupuncture has a balancing, homeostatic effect. The same point can be used in the event of under- and over-functioning. For example the Large Intestine point can be used to treat both constipation and diarrhoea.

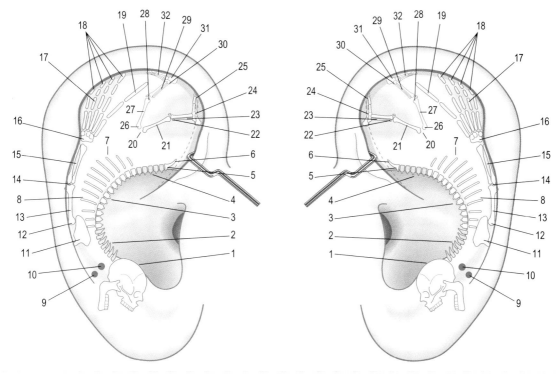

Figure 7.1 The skeleton.

1. Cranium
2. Cervical Vertebrae, C1–C7
3. Thoracic Vertebrae, Th1–Th2
4. Lumbar Vertebrae, L1–L5
5. Sacrum
6. Coccyx
7. Rib Bone
8. Sternum
9. Collar Bone (F)
10. Collar Bone (C)
11. Shoulder Blade
12. Shoulder Joint
13. Upper Arm
14. Elbow
15. Underarm
16. Wrist
17. Hand
18. Fingers
19. Thumb
20. Hip Joint (F), Pelvic Girdle
21. Thigh (F)
22. Knee (F)
23. Lower Leg (F)
24. Foot (F)
25. Toes (F)
26. Hip Joint (C)
27. Thigh (C)
28. Knee (C)
29. Lower Leg (C)
30. Ankle (C)
31. Foot (C)
32. Toes (C)

The locomotor system

The locomotor system is comprised of components of the skeleton and muscula-ture. A little upside-down human being is reflected in the ear. The skull and most of its related parts (the cranium, brain, eyes, etc) are to be found in the earlobe. The backbone is reflected along the antihelix and its lower leg. The arm is reflected in the scaphoid fossa, the leg on the upper leg of the antihelix or in fossa triangularis.

Cranium (1) (see Fig. 7.1)

Where is it? The zone corresponding to the cranium fills the antitragus.

Indications? Pain or malfunctioning in the equivalent body part. In the same zone are points corresponding to the central nervous system, for example the points Brain, Hypothalamus, Brainstem and Thalamus. (The lobes of the brain have a larger reflex zone than the cranium so that it covers a greater part of the earlobe.)

Backbone — Cervical Vertebrae, Thoracic Vertebrae, Thorax, Lower Back, Small of the Back, Coccyx (2–6) (see Fig. 7.1, page 71)

Where is it? The points for the seven cervical vertebrae, the 12 thoracic vertebrae, the five lumbar vertebrae, the sacrum and the coccyx lie in a row along the edge of the antihelix, according to the order they have in the body. Between Cranium and the reflex point for the first cervical vertebra there is a groove, LM 14. So the point for the first cervical vertebra is just above LM 14, while that for the first thoracic vertebra can be found where an extension of the helix root should meet the antihelix (LM 15). The point for the first lumbar vertebra lies on the edge of the antihelix's lower leg, near Kidney (C). The Sacrum and Coccyx lie under the edge of the helix.

When you search for the reflex point to a vertebra with a pen resembling a screwdriver, use the flat end of the pen to palpate it. Draw it slowly with equal pressure along the edge of the antihelix. The patient will grimace or tell you that it is sore when you pass over the zone which is the reflex point for the vertebra that is in pain.

If the pain derives from the vertebrae, the sore point will very often be in a zone on the inner side of the antihelix, close to the edge. The reflex points for each disc are near those for the respective vertebrae, on the wall, closer to the concha. If the pain comes from the musculature, the active point will usually be on the other side of the antihelix facing towards the scaphoid fossa. This part of the antihelix is called 'Paravertebral Muscles and Ligaments' (see Fig. 7.2). Here you'll find the points called Neck, Chest, Buttocks, Abdomen and Thorax.

Indications: Pain or malfunctioning in the corresponding part of the locomotor system, or in the part of the body innervated by the nerve that runs from the particular vertebra.

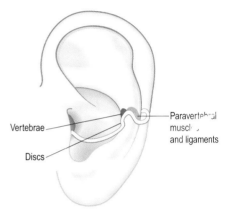

Figure 7.2 Cross-section of the antihelix with the zones that correspond to the vertebrae, the discs and the thoracic muscles and ligaments.

Ribs (Thorax, Chest) (7) (see Fig. 7.1, page 71)

Where is it? On the antihelix. The reflex zone for every rib bone stretches from the reflex point for the vertebra to which the rib is fastened and out over the antihelix.

Indications? Pain in the rib bone, intercostal neuralgia. Used also for angina pectoris, asthma, coughing and hiccoughing.

Sternum (Breast Bone) (8) (see Fig. 7.1, page 71)

Where is it? On the antihelix.

Indications? Pain or other malfunctioning in the corresponding body part.

Collar Bone (F), Collar Bone (C) (Clavicle) (9–10) (see Fig. 7.1, page 71)

Where is it? Collar bone (F) lies on the antihelix, on a level with the apex of the antitragus and the cervical vertebrae. Collar Bone (C) lies a little lower down, in the scaphoid fossa.

Indications? Pain or malfunctioning of the corresponding body part.

Shoulder Blade (Scapula, Deltoid Muscle Point) (11) (see Fig. 7.1, page 71)

Where is it? In the lower part of the scaphoid fossa. The point can lie on a level with, or right below the level of the helix root, above Collar Bone (C), under Shoulder Joint.

Indications? Pain or malfunctioning of the corresponding body part.

Shoulder Joint, Upper Arm, Elbow, Lower Arm, Wrist, Hand, Fingers and Thumb (12–19) (see Fig. 7.1, page 71)

Where is it? The points for the arm and hand are in the scaphoid fossa. Shoulder Joint lies on a level with the helix root where an extension of the helix root would cross the scaphoid fossa. In the same order of the body parts they represent, there then follow the point for Upper Arm, Elbow (which lies on a level with the lower leg of the antihelix), Lower Arm, Wrist (which lies on a level with Darwin's tubercle) and Hand. The zone for the Upper Arm is half as long as the zone for the Lower Arm. The Lower Arm is as big as the Hand.

The hand is represented with the four fingers uppermost in the scaphoid fossa. Sometimes the fingers reach up under the helix so that the fingertips are concealed under its edge. The Thumb stretches up on the upper leg of the antihelix where it meets the Big Toe (C).

Indications? Pain or some other malfunction in the corresponding part of the body.

The Pelvic Girdle (Pelvic Bone, Hip Joint (F), Pelvic Cavity, Sacroiliac Joint) (20) (see Fig. 7.1, page 71)

Where is it? In the bottom part of the tip of the cavity of the fossa triangularis, under and close to Shen Men.

Indications? Pelvic pain, symphysis pubis dysfunction (SPD), low back pain, painful menstruation, pelvic weakness, endometriosis, prostate trouble.

Hip Joint, Thigh, Knee, Lower Leg, Ankle, Foot and Toes (all both (F) and (C)) (20–32) (see Fig. 7.1, page 71)

Where is it? The body's lower extremity is drawn in differently on the French and Chinese point maps. The Leg (F) has the hip at the tip of the fossa triangularis, right under Shen Men, and the leg stretched out in the cavity. As on the body, the hip is connected to the thigh bone, the knee, lower leg, ankle and the feet in that order. Ankle (F) is located near the helix. Heel (F) is depicted pointing downwards and Toes (F) points up towards the apex. Sometimes Heel (F), Ankle (F) and Toes (F) are to be found under the edge of the helix. Heel (C) lies near Coccyx, and the Achilles tendon is shown near the reflex zone for the Sacrum.

Hip (C) is to be found higher up on the helix comparable with Hip (F), where the antihelix divides into its lower and upper legs. On the Chinese map, from the Hip point the leg stretches upwards along the upper leg of the antihelix with Foot (C) close to, or under the edge of the helix. Toes (C) points backwards and Big Toe (C) almost meets the Thumb.

Indications? Pain or some other malfunction in the corresponding part of the body.

Neck (Back of the Head, Occipital Masterpoint, Occipital Triggerpoint, Occiput, Occipital Skull, Atlas of Head, Pad Point) (see Fig. 7.3)

Near the reflex point for the first cervical vertebra lies a point which is generally considered a good place to treat all painful conditions of the back. It also influences several functions. It is called the Neck point but sometimes too Back of the Head because it also corresponds to the rear part of the skull. Neck is both a reflex and functional point.

Where is it? Near LM 14, which is between the antitragus and the antihelix, 2–3 mm below the edge of the antihelix, in the direction of Jerome's point.

Indications? The point is analgesic, calming and anti-inflammatory. It is used for treatment of sciatica, pains in the neck and the whole backbone, nerve pain in the face, the ribs, sleeping problems, nightmares, anxiety, tense headaches, aching at the back of the head and neck, acute migraine, nausea, dizziness. Used as a prophylactic in cases of travel sickness.

According to traditional Chinese medicine (TCM), treatment of the Neck point removes wind and heat.

Neck muscles (34) (see Fig. 7.3)

Where? On the antihelix, in the zone 'paravertebrale muscles and ligaments' in the same level as the reflex points for the neck vertebrae.

Indications? Pain or other dysfunction in the corresponding body part.

Breast 1 (Mammae)(35) (see Fig. 7.3)

Where is it? On the antihelix, above the level of the helix root and on a level with Th5. The point can be found on the ridge of the antihelix, or on the part of antihelix facing towards the scaphoid fossa.

Indications? Pain or malfunctioning of the corresponding part of the body, for example premenstrual tension, retention of milk and other problems with lactation.

Breast 2 (Mammary Gland) (36) (see Fig. 7.3)

The breast also has a hormonal point. Breast 2 is described on page 87.

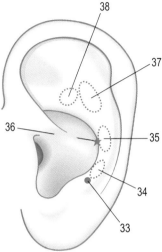

Figure 7.3 Reflex zones for some of the soft parts of the locomotor system, and the Neck point, in the zone called 'Paravertebral Muscles and Ligaments'.

33. Neck point
34. Neck Muscles
35. Breast 1 (the soft breast)
36. Breast 2 (control point for breast glands)
37. Abdominal Muscles
38. Buttocks

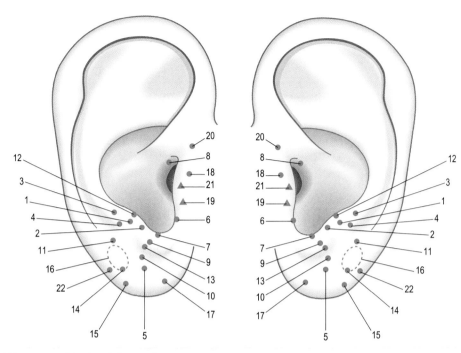

Figure 7.4 The zones of the head, face and sensory organs.

1. Temple
2. Forehead
3. Neck
4. Crown of the Head
5. Eye
6. Eye 1
7. Eye 2
8. Mouth
9. Upper Palate
10. Lower Palate
11. Jaw/Salivary Gland 1
12. Salivary Gland 2
13. Tongue (C)
14. Tongue (F)
15. Lips
16. Zone for Cheek/Face
17. Inner Nose (F)
18. External Nose (C)
19. Inner Nose
20. External Ear
21. Inner Ear (F)
22. Inner Ear (C)

Abdomen (37) (see Fig. 7.3, page 74)

Where is it? On the upper part of the antihelix, before it divides into its upper and lower legs, above Breast 1.
  Indications? Pain or malfunction in the abdominal muscles.

Buttocks (38) (see Fig. 7.3, page 74)

Where is it? Close to Hip joint (C) but further forward, on the lower leg of the antihelix.
  Indications? Pain or other dysfunction in the corresponding body part.

The head, face and sense organs

Cranium (see Fig. 7.1, page 71)

Temple (Tai Yang) (1) (see Fig. 7.4)

Where is it? On the antitragus, between Forehead and Neck, near Brain.

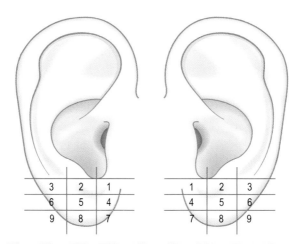

Figure 7.5 The earlobe is divided into squares. Some points are indicated according to the square in which they are located.

Indications? Headache in the temples, migraine, dizziness, tinnitus. Calming. According to TCM, Temple corresponds to the body acupuncture point Tai Yang and removes wind.

Forehead (Frontal Sinus, Frontal Skull point) (2) (see Fig. 7.4, page 75)

Where is it? In the forward part of the antitragus.
Indications? Anxiety, headache in the forehead, sinus inflammation, sleeping problems, dizziness.

Neck (3) (see Fig. 7.4 This point is described on page 71, page 74)

This point is described on page 71.

Crown of the Head (Vertex, Apex of Head) (4) (see Fig. 7.4, page 75)

Where is it? In the lower, rear quadrant of the antitragus, under Neck.
Indications? Headache at the crown of the head, dizziness.

Eye (Retina, Master Sensorial) (5) (see Fig. 7.4, page 75)

The eye has three reflex points in the ear: Eye, Eye 1 and Eye 2.
Where is it? One of the eye points, which is simply called Eye, is the point which is most often used to make a hole in the ear for wearing ear-rings. It lies in the centre of the lobe, in square number 5 (see Fig. 7.5). In many cultures it is a tradition to make a hole in the ear of baby girls at a very early age. Nogier had a theory that this was because some venereal diseases could be transmitted from the mother to the baby's eyes during childbirth. By pricking the point Eye the baby's eyes would be protected from infection.
Pirates wore a gold ring in one ear because, according to legend, this gave them better sight when looking out for ships to plunder. According to some texts, sight is improved if a ring is put in the Eye point of the dominant ear.
Indications? See Eye 1 and Eye 2.

Eye 1 (Glaucoma) and Eye 2 (Astigmatism) (6–7) (see Fig. 7.4, page 75)

Where are they? Two other points for the eye lie one on each side of the incisura interagica.

Indications? All three eye points are used to treat ocular problems, such as disturbed eyesight, irritation, bloodshot eyes, dry eye syndrome, eye inflammation, headache behind the eyes etc. (For tics around the eye, see functional point Tics, page 124.) Eye 1, which lies in front of the incisura intertragica, is sometimes called Glaucoma and Eye 2 is known in Chinese texts as Astigmatism, which suggests that the Chinese thought the two points had different effects.

Mouth (8) (see Fig. 7.4, page 75)

Where is it? In the cavum concha, high up, near the external ear canal and the helix root.

Indications? Problems in the mouth, ulcers, stomatitis, facial paralysis. Also used during slimming to diminish hunger, and in helping smokers to quit.

According to TCM, Mouth reduces 'fire in the heart'.

Palate, Upper and Lower (9–10) (see Fig. 7.4, page 75)

Where is it? The reflex point for the palate in the lower jaw is in square number 2 of the earlobe. The reflex point for the palate in the upper jaw is at the borderline between the second and fifth square of the earlobe.

Indications? Pain, sores, infections in the corresponding part of the body.

Jaw Joint, Jaw, Upper and Lower Jaw (11) (see Fig. 7.4, page 75) (Temporomandibular Joint (TMJ), Maxillary Point, Lower Jaw, Upper Jaw, Teeth, Antidepression 2, Salivary Gland, Parotid Gland, Lips)

Where is it? The reflex points for both the upper and lower jaw are in the third square of the earlobe, a few millimetres from one another, according to — among other authorities — the World Health Organisation. However, in certain Chinese texts both the upper and lower jaw points are in the lobe's second square.

Indications? Toothache, other painful conditions in the mouth, problems with the jaw joint, the grinding together of teeth, trigeminal neuralgia. For pain relief during tooth extraction or filling. (See also Toothache, page 112.)

Salivary Gland 1 and 2 (Parotis, Parotid Gland, Jaw Joint, Jaw, Upper and Lower Jaw) (11–12) (see Fig. 7.4, page 75)

The parotid gland is the salivary gland under the ear. Two points have been designated this name.

Where are they? Salivary Gland 1 is in the rear part of the earlobe, in the scaphoid fossa, in square number 3, near Jaw. Salivary gland 2 is at the apex of the antitragus, close to Asthma 2.

Indications? Dryness in the mouth, mumps, infections in the salivary gland.

Tongue (C) and (F) (13–14) (see Fig. 7.4, page 75)

Where are they? Tongue (C) is in the second square of the earlobe, above Eye. Tongue (F) is in the sixth square of the earlobe, behind Eye, diagonally under Jaw. (There is also a large zone for the tongue at Nogier's reflex map, on the helix, starting at Darwin's tubercle and ending at the apex.)

Indications? Problems with the tongue, the throat and with speech.

According to TCM, Tongue reduces 'fire in the heart'.

Lips (15) (see Fig. 7.4, page 75)

Where is it? In the ninth square of the earlobe, close to and behind LM 7.

Indications? Dry, cracked lips and ulcers.

Cheek/Face (16) (see Fig. 7.4, page 75)

Where is it? On the earlobe, in a large oval zone on the border between the fifth and the sixth square, behind Eye which lies in the centre of the lobe, in front of Inner Ear (C).

Indications? Facial paralysis, trigeminal neuralgia, acne, mumps and other symptoms of the cheek.

Nose

There is one point for the outer part of the nose (External Nose) and two for the inside (Inner Nose). Inner Nose corresponds primarily to the mucous membrane and the functions of the nose. External Nose corresponds to the skin of the nose.

Inner Nose (F) (Olfactory Nerve, First Cranial Nerve, Olfactive Point) (17) (see Fig. 7.4, page 75)

Where is it? On the earlobe, in square four.

Indications? Problems with smell sensations.

External Nose (C) (18) (see Fig. 7.4, page 75)

Where is it? In a groove in front of the upper curve of the tragus, on a level with the external ear canal.

Indications? Red nose, acne rosacea, pimples, sunburn.

Inner Nose (Nasal Cavity) (19) (see Fig. 7.4, page 75)

Where is it? On the inside of the tragus (subtragus).

Indications? Nasal congestion, nasal catarrh, rhinitis, sinusitis, epistaxis (nose bleeding).

Sinus

Where is it? For frontal sinus, look for the active point in or directly under Forehead. For the sinuses of the jaw look for the active point close to the zones for Inner Nose and Jaw.

Indications? Sinusitis.

External Ear (Auricle, Pinna) (20) (see Fig. 7.4, page 75)

Where is it? In the upper part of the groove in front of the tragus, near the ascending part of helix, above External Nose (C), between Frustration and Vitality.

    Indications? Tinnitus and other hearing difficulties, infection, external otitis, signs of cartilage infection and other damage to the external ear.

Inner Ear (F) (Auditory Nerve, CN VII, Eighth Cranial Nerve, Cochleovestibularis Nerve) (21) (see Fig. 7.4, page 75)

Where is it? On the inside of the tragus (subtragus), above Inner Nose.

    Indications? Ear symptoms such as hearing loss, infection, tinnitus, dizziness, balance problems. (See also functional point Auditory Zone, page 124.)

Inner Ear (C) (Balance, Middle Ear, Auditory Line, Auditory Zone) (22) (see Fig. 7.4, page 75)

Where is it? Inner Ear (C) is to be found in the sixth square of the earlobe, behind Eye and Cheek.

    Indications? Ear symptoms such as hearing loss, infection, tinnitus, dizziness, balance problems. (See too functional point Auditory Zone, page 124.)

    According to TCM, Ear strengthens the kidney's yin and reduces yang in the liver.

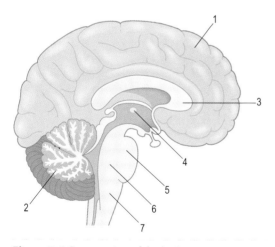

Figure 7.6 Cross-section of the brain.

1. Cerebrum
2. Cerebellum
3. Corpus callosum
4. Thalamus
5. Pons
6. Medulla oblongata
7. Spinal cord

The nervous system

In a zone that covers both the inside and the outside of the antitragus and goes down to LM 14, there are a series of points that correspond with different parts of the brain. Certain point maps note a series of points on the antitragus with names connected to the various parts and functions of the brain. However, I have chosen to regard this part of the ear as a zone which corresponds to the whole of the brain and to name three specific points in this zone: Brain on the outside of the antitragus; and Thalamus and Hypothalamus on the inside. At the crossover between the antitragus and the antihelix, close to LM 14, you'll find Cerebellum and Brainstem. In a zone running inside and parallel with the antihelix on the wall of the concha, the sympathetic trunk is depicted along with the reflex points of several nerves. So too the Zone with Control Points for the Hormonal Glands which influences hormonal activity in the various organs. Still more reflex points for the nervous system are included.

    The cranium has a smaller zone than the brain, see page 71.

    See Figs. 7.6 and 7.7.

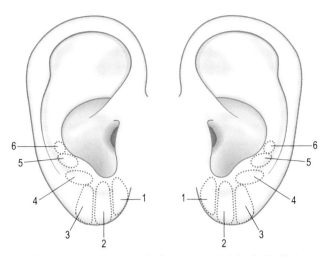

Figure 7.7 Reflex zones for the lobes of the brain and the cerebellum.

1. Prefrontal Lobe
2. Frontal Lobe
3. Parietal Lobe
4. Temple Lobe
5. Occipital Lobe
6. Cerebellum

Brain (in this zone are points called Encephalon [Latin for 'brain'], Limbic system, Cerebral, Depression, Excitation, Middle Border, Nervus, Pain Control Point, Asthma and Ding Shuan [which means 'soothes asthma'], Sun Point) (1) (see Fig. 7.8, page 81)

Where is it? In a zone which covers the antitragus and the lobe, there are several points corresponding to the various parts of the brain. The Lobes of the Brain are to be found on the earlobe (see Fig. 7.7). The reflex zone for the frontal lobe lies furthest forward, followed by the parietal, temporal and occipital lobes. Choose active points in the zone.

The point called Brain is situated in the middle of the base line of the antitragus, directly across from Thalamus, which lies on the inside of the antitragus.

Indications? Damage, pain or other malfunctioning. Acute and chronic headache, including migraine. Emotional imbalance, depression, poor memory, insomnia and dizziness.

In the 1970s the research team in Nanking described the point's function as hormonal. They thought it corresponded to the pituitary gland and recommended it be treated in cases of poor growth, asthma, menstruation, sleeping difficulties and bedwetting.

Thalamus (Pain Control Point, Brain, Cerebral Master Point, Dermis, Excitement) (2) (see Fig. 7.8, page 81)

Where is it? Thalamus is both a reflex point and a functional point with considerable systemic effects. It is situated low down on the inside wall of the antitragus, where the wall meets the bottom of the concha. On the inside of the antitragus

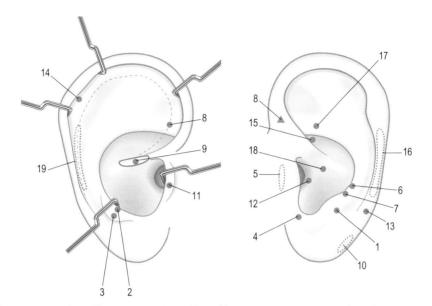

Figure 7.8 Points for the central nervous system plus Point Zero and San Jiao.

1. Brain
2. Thalamus
3. Hypothalamus
4. Pineal Gland
5. Corpus Callosum
6. Cerebellum
7. Brainstem
8. Sympathetic Autonomic Point
9. Solar Plexus/Point Zero
10. Trigeminal Zone
11. Auditory Nerve
12. Vagus Nerve 1
13. Vagus Nerve 2
14. Lesser Occipital Nerve
15. Hypogastric Plexus
16. Spinal Cord
17. Sciatica
18. Bronchopulmonary Plexus
19. Vegetative Groove

you'll sometimes find a crease from the apex to the concha. Thalamus lies at the bottom of this indentation. Look for active points in the zone and treat them.

Indications? Acute and chronic pain, disturbances in the central nervous system, after stroke, and disorders in the digestive, hormonal and urogenital systems, in cases of high blood pressure, sleeping problems, sweating, swellings, anxiety and shock.

Thalamus is one of the most important of the pain-relieving points in ear acupuncture. Thalamus regulates activity in the cerebral cortex and can be used on occasions when such activity is too high or too low. According to Oleson (2003), Thalamus corresponds to the whole diencephalon, including the thalamus and hypothalamus. The Thalamus point is thought to reduce acute and chronic pain by activating the thalamus gate in the supraspinal pain inhibition system.

The point can be used to treat the types of tinnitus and bedwetting that, according to TCM, are caused by weak kidney qi. According to TCM, the kidneys are responsible for the development and efficient functioning of the central nervous system and the brain. Thalamus is also used to treat neurasthenia, exhaustion depression, depression and schizophrenia.

Thalamus is one of what Oleson (2003) calls 'primary masterpoints'.

Hypothalamus (Vegetative Point 2, Subcortex, Grey Matter) (3) (see Fig. 7.8, page 81)

Sometimes Hypothalamus is given as a specific point. In other books it is counted together with Thalamus. Like Thalamus it is both a reflex point and a functional point, with considerable systemic effect.

Where is it? On the inside of the antitragus, a few millimetres above Thalamus, between Thalamus and the apex of the antitragus.

Indications? Hypothalamus regulates the autonomous nervous system, which in turn regulates, among other things, body warmth, sleep and wakefulness, blood pressure, breathing, hunger, liquid balance, perspiration, hormonal activity and sexuality. The Hypothalamus point is considered to have a homeostatic effect and is recommended in cases of imbalance in any of the autonomous functions, in acute and chronic painful inflammation and stress.

Pineal Gland (E-point, E3, Epiphysis) (4) (see Fig. 7.8, page 81)

Where is it? In the hormonal zone, on the lowest part of the tragus, near Eye 1 and Aggression.

Indications? The pineal gland releases melatonin which influences the body's daily cycle. Its point can be treated in cases of disturbed rhythm, jet lag and sleeping disorders.

Corpus Callosum (5) (see Fig. 7.8, page 81)

Where is it? In a long zone in front of the tragus, in the groove where the cartilage comes to an end.

Indications? Corpus callosum links together the two halves of the brain and has a function related to laterality (see Ch. 5, Explanatory models for acupuncture) and balancing the work of the two halves. This point can be treated in cases of symptoms linked to disturbance in laterality (for example, bedwetting, stammering and learning difficulties).

Cerebellum (6) (see Fig. 7.8, page 81)

Where is it? Close to the groove that divides the antitragus from the antihelix, LM 14, on the ridge of the antihelix.

Indications? Dizziness, balancing and coordination difficulties, intention tremor, nystagmus.

Brainstem (Medulla Oblongata, Vomiting, Kinetosis, Antiemetica, Nausea) (7) (see Fig. 7.8, page 81)

Where is it? On upper rear of the antitragus, close to LM 14. Brainstem also has a reflex point on the descending helix, in the bottom part of the zone for the spinal cord.

Indications? Damage or malfunctioning of the brainstem or of the brain in general. Influences body temperature, breathing, cardiac activity, headaches, multiple sclerosis, vomiting, nausea and travel sickness.

Sympathetic Autonomic Point (Sympaticus, Autonomous Point, Vegetativum) (8) (see Fig. 7.8, page 81)

Where is it? Sympathetic Autonomic Point is both a reflex and a functional point with considerable systemic effect. It lies under the edge of the helix and is invisible when looking straight ahead at the ear. The needle should be aligned parallel with the lower leg of the antihelix, laid under the edge of the helix and inserted at the bottom of the crease under the helix where the lower leg of the antihelix comes to an end.

Indications? Malfunctioning of the internal organs, anxiety, involuntary perspiration, night sweat, pain.

Sympathetic Autonomic Point balances the activity in both the sympathetic and parasympathetic nervous systems and is used when there are disturbances in them. In so doing the internal imbalance is reduced and there is a beneficial effect on various internal organs. Sympathetic Autonomic Point is thought to improve blood circulation, correct irregular and rapid heart beat and to soothe angina. Sympathetic Autonomic Point has a relaxing effect on the internal organs and has antispasmodic properties (combats cramp), for example in cases of colic pain, renal colic and gallstone attacks. It has a very relaxing and soothing effect in the event of stress. It is a strong painkiller and is used during acupuncture anaesthetic. According to TCM, it gives nourishment to yin and supports yang.

Sympathetic Autonomic Point is one of the five points Oleson (1998) describes as 'primary masterpoints'. It is also one of the five NADA points.[2]

Solar Plexus (Point Zero, Celiac Plexus, Thoracic Splanchnic Nerves, Abdominal Brain) (9) (see Fig. 7.8, page 81)

Both a reflex and functional point.

Where is it? Solar Plexus occupies a zone on the helix root. Point Zero lies in the front section of the zone and Stomach in its rear section. Sometimes Solar Plexus is marked as a smaller point in or close to Point Zero.

Indications? Symptoms connected with the abdomen and its organs, anxiety.

Trigeminal Zone (CN V, Fifth Cranial Nerve, Trigeminal Nerve, Trigeminal Nucleus) (10) (see Fig. 7.8, page 81)

The fifth cranial nerve is called the trigeminal. One branch of it goes to the region around the eyes, another to the upper jaw and a third to the lower jaw.

Where is it? On the earlobe, at the rear edge of the sixth and ninth squares.

Indications? Trigeminal neuralgia (with bleeding technique), toothache.

Auditory nerve (CN VIII, Eighth Cranial Nerve, Inner Ear (F), Cochleovestibularis Nerve) (11) (see Fig. 7.8, page 81)

Where is it? On the inside of the tragus (subtragus), near Inner Nose.

Indications? Symptoms connected to the ear, such as reduced hearing, infection, tinnitus, dizziness, balance problems. (See too functional point Auditory Zone, page 124.)

Olfactory Nerve (Inner Nose (F), CN 1, First Cranial Nerve, Olfactive Point)

See Inner Nose (F), page 78.

---

[2] NADA is a standardised form of ear acupuncture used to fight drug addiction, see Ch. 13, NADA – using ear acupuncture to fight addiction.

Vagus Nerve 1 and 2 (CN X, Tenth Cranial Nerve) (12–13) (see Fig. 7.8, page 81)

The vagus nerve is the largest parasympathetic nerve.

Where is it? The vagus nerve has two reflex points. Vagus Nerve 1 is on the bottom of the concha in front of the external ear canal, above the functional point San Jiao, which is considered to have a similar function (see page 117). Vagus Nerve 2 is on the helix, level with the incisura intertragica, in the zone for Medulla Oblongata.

Indications? Symptoms connected with the autonomous nervous system such as sweating, arrhythmias, indigestion, heartburn, intestinal and urinary troubles, diarrhoea, anxiety.

Accessory Nerve (CN XI, Eleventh Cranial Nerve) (see Fig. 7.9)

The accessory nerve has one branch that connects it to the vagus nerve while another goes to the thorax and shoulder musculature. It is a motor nerve which acts on the sternocleidomastoideus and trapezius muscles.

Where is it? On the rear of the helix, at a level with incisura intertragica.
Indications? Torticollis, wryneck.

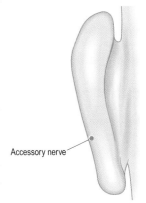

Accessory nerve

Figure 7.9 Accessory nerve.

Lesser Occipital Nerve (Minor Occipital Nerve, Wind Stream) (14) (see Fig. 7.8, page 81)

Where is it? On the inside of the helix, approximately 2 mm above LM 3, the groove that borders the upper edge of Darwin's tubercle.

Indications? Pain, migraine, neckache, paralysis on one side of the body and other consequences of stroke, dizziness. Calming.

Hypogastric Plexus (Omega 1, Inferior Mesenteric Ganglion, Lumbosacral Splanchnic Nerve, Mercury Toxicity E1), (15) (see Fig. 7.8, page 81)

Where is it? In the cymba concha, beneath and in front of the Urinary Bladder and between it and Small Intestine/Large Intestine on a level with Weather and External Genitalia (F).

Indications? Influences the autonomous nervous system. Used when there are problems with urination or with the functioning of the intestines. Overload of amalgam, and other environmental factors.

The Reticular System

See Master Oscillation, Ch. 8, Functional points (page 110).

Spinal Cord (16) (see Fig. 7.8, page 81)

Where is it? On the outside of the helix, in a zone that starts above Brainstem, on a level with LM 14, and that ends at Darwin's tubercle. In the bottom part of this long, slim zone lie reflex points which correspond to the portion of the spinal cord passing through the cervical vertebrae, above those reflex points which correspond to the spinal cord at thoracic vertebrae level and near Darwin's tubercle reflex points that correspond to the spinal cord at lumbar vertebrae level. On the rear of the helix is a corresponding zone used to treat motor problems.

Indications? Slipped disc, shingles, neuralgia.

Sciatica (Lumbago, Sciatic Nerve, Sacroiliac Joint) (17) (see Fig. 7.8, page 81)

Where is it? Sciatica lies on the lower leg of the antihelix, close to and just above the points that correspond to lumbar vertebrae 4 and 5, between Sympathetic Autonomic Point and Buttocks. (It is this point that throughout history has been treated by using a small red-hot instrument to make a burn mark and ease the pain of sciatica.)

Indications? Sciatic pain, lumbago.

Bronchopulmonary Plexus (18) (see Fig. 7.8, page 81)

Where is it? In the upper part of the cavum concha, above Heart (C), under Stomach. Coincides with Upper Lung.

Indications? Bronchial spasms as in asthma.

Vegetative Groove (19) (see Fig. 7.8, page 81)

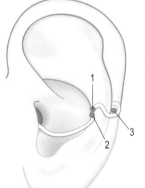

Where is it? In a thin, oblong zone under the edge of the helix is a zone which corresponds to the sensory nerves. The Vegetative Groove starts between the lower and upper leg of the antitragus and ends in the tail of the helix.

Indications? Segment-related symptoms, pain, neuralgia.

Sympathetic Trunk (Paravertebral Chain of Sympathetic Ganglia, Postganglionic Sympathetic Nerves) (see Figs 7.10 and 7.11, pages 85 and 86)

Where is it? In a zone along the wall of the concha, parallel with and closer to the concha than the zone for the spinal vertebrae and discs and the one with control points for the hormonal glands. In the Sympathetic Trunk zone are to be found points called Superior Cervical Ganglion, Middle Cervical Ganglion (also called Muscle Relaxation and Cardiac Plexus) and Inferior Cervical Ganglion (Ganglion Stellatum).

Figure 7.10 Cross-section of the antihelix with the zone containing the reflex points for the sympathetic trunk, the zone with Control Points for the Hormonal Glands and with the Vegetative groove.

1. Zone with Control Points for the Hormonal Glands.
2. Zone Corresponding to the Sympathetic Trunk.
3. Vegetative Groove.

Superior Cervical Ganglion (1) (see Fig. 7.11, page 86)

Where is it? In the Sympathetic Trunk zone on a level with cervical vertebra C1.

Indications? A regulatory effect on that part of the sympathetic trunk which starts at the neck. Influences the flow of blood, tears, saliva and sweating on the face.

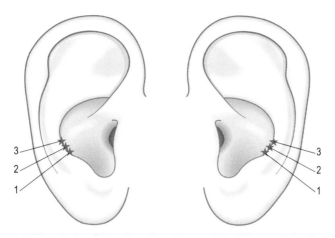

Figure 7.11 Three points in the reflex zone for the Sympathetic Trunk.

1. Superior Cervical Ganglion
2. Middle Cervical Ganglion/Cardiac Plexus/Muscle Relaxation
3. Inferior Cervical Ganglion/Ganglion Stellatum

Cardiac Plexus (Muscle Relaxation, Middle Cervical Plexus, Middle Cervical Ganglion , Wonder Point, Marvellous Point, Jisong) (2) (see Fig. 7.11)

Where is it? In the zone representing the sympathetic trunk, on a level with the reflex points for cervical vertebrae C3–C5. On the wall of the concha, where the extension of the helix root's lower part meets the antihelix. Here I use the name Cardiac Plexus to show its connection to the nervous system but elsewhere in the book the point will be called Muscle Relaxation.

Indications? Muscular tension, stress, pain. Relaxes muscles in the whole body. Reduces activity in the sympathetic nervous system, lowers blood pressure. Regulates the activity of the heart, blood pressure and the flow of blood to the face. Helps when there is a tendency to faint during periods of anxiety. May also be used in operations where acupuncture is employed as an anaesthetic to get muscles to relax.

Ganglion Stellatum (Inferior Cervical Ganglion, Shoulder Master Point, Stellate Ganglion, Cervical-Thoracic Ganglia) (3) (see Fig. 7.11)

Where is it? In the Sympathetic Trunk zone, on a level with the reflex points for vertebrae C7/Th1.

Indications? Unilateral headache, neuralgia in the neck region, whiplash, shoulder pain, nausea.

Zone of Nervous Control Points of Hormonal Glands

Where is it? The Zone with Control Points for the Hormonal Glands lies parallel with the reflex zone for the Backbone, on the wall of the concha, between the reflex

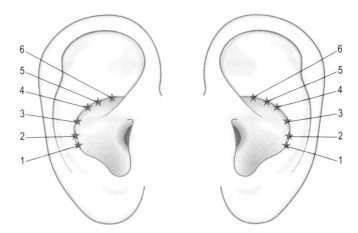

Figure 7.12 Points in the Zone with Control Points for the Hormonal Glands.

1. Parathyroid Gland
2. Thyroid Gland 2
3. Breast 2
4. Thymus
5. Pancreas 2
6. Adrenal Gland 1

zone for the Vertebrae and the reflex zone for Sympathetic Trunk (see Fig. 7.10). We shall now detail the points in this zone, which are Parathyroid, Thyroid Gland 2, Breast 2, Thymus, Pancreas and Adrenal Gland 1.

Parathyroid Gland (Endocrine Parathyroid Gland Point) (1) (see Fig. 7.12)

Where is it? In the Zone with Control Points for the Hormonal Glands, on a level with the reflex points for cervical vertebrae C5–C6.

Indications? Dysfunctions of the parathyroid gland. Muscle cramps when the calcium metabolism is disturbed.

Thyroid Gland 2, hormonal point (Hormonal Thyroid Gland, Endocrine Thyroid Gland, Thyroidea Plexus) (2) (see Fig. 7.12)

Where is it? In the Zone of Control Points for the Hormonal Glands, in level with the reflex points for Cervical Vertebrae C6–C7, right above Parathyroid Gland. (There is another reflex point for the thyroid, Thyroid Gland 1, see page 91.)

Indications? Regulates both over- and underfunctioning of the thyroid gland.

Breast 2 (Mammary Gland) (3) (see Fig. 7.12)

Where is it? In the Zone with Control Points for the Hormonal Glands, on a level with the reflex point for Th5, between the hormonal points for Thyroid Gland 2 and Thymus. Despite the fact that the female breast is not an endocrinal gland, it has a control point in this zone.

There is another point called Breast 1, located on the antihelix at a level with the reflex point for cervical vertebra Th5, see page 74.

Indications? Problems with breastfeeding, too little milk, tense breasts in connection with premenstrual tension.

Thymus, hormonal point (Thymus Gland Point, Thymic Plexus) (4) (see Fig. 7.12, page 87)

Where is it? In the Zone of Control Points for the hormonal glands, between Liver and Kidney (C), also between Pancreas and Breast 2.

Indications? Reduced immune defence, for example as concerns allergies, infections, autoimmune illnesses. An important functional point with anti-inflammatory, antirheumatic and antiallergic effect.

Pancreas 2, hormonal point (Endocrine Pancreas, Insulin Point) (5) (see Fig. 7.12, page 87)

Where is it? In the Zone of Control Points for the Hormonal Glands, between Thymus and Adrenal Gland 2.

Indications? Problems with the pancreas, hypoglycaemia.

Adrenal Gland 1, hormonal point (ACTH, Glandula Suprarenalis, Cortisone) (6) (see Fig. 7.12, page 87)

The adrenal gland regulates the hormones. ACTH is short for adrenocorticotropic hormone. It is produced in the frontal lobe of the pituitary gland and governs the production of cortisol in the cortex of the adrenal gland, and thus the amount of cortisol in the body. The hormonal point for the adrenal gland is thought to generate an effect similar to cortisone. (There are two more points called Adrenal Gland, see page 101).

Where is it? In the Zone of Control Points for the Hormonal Glands, above Kidney (C).

Indications? Pain, allergies and inflammation, rheumatic aches, skin complaints, itching, asthma, anxiety, phobias, exhaustion syndromes, stress.

The throat and respiratory system

The nose and mouth are openings for the respiratory tract. This carries air into the body — down the larynx and trachea to the bronchi and then to the lungs (Fig. 7.13). The lungs control the vitally important function of exchanging oxygen and carbon dioxide. The tonsils are part of the throat's lymph system. In the ear there are reflex points for all these organs, from Mouth to Lung, in a row on the cavum concha.

The points for Nose and Mouth (1) (see Fig. 7.14) are described on pages 77–79 under the heading 'The head, face and sensory organs'.

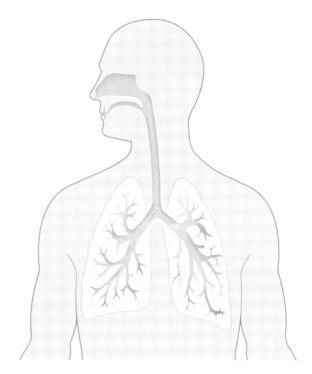

Figure 7.13 The respiratory system.

Throat (C) and Throat (F) (Pharynx) (2–3) (see Fig. 7.14, page 90)

Where are they? Throat (C) is on the upper part of the inside of the tragus (subtragus), directly above Larynx (C). Throat (F) is in the cavum concha, between Mouth and Larynx.

Indications? Pharyngitis, hoarseness, tonsillitis and other throat problems.

Larynx (C) and Larynx (F) (4–5) (see Fig. 7.14, page 90)

Where are they? Larynx (C) is on the upper part of the inside of the tragus (subtragus), directly under Throat (C). Larynx (F) is in the cavum concha, near Mouth.

Indications? Laryngitis, sore throat, difficulties in swallowing.

Windpipe (Trachea) (6) (see Fig. 7.14, page 90)

Where is it? At the bottom of the cavum concha, in the lung zone, between Heart (C), Bronchi and Mouth.

Indications? Coughing, sore throat, hoarseness, asthma, phlegm.

Bronchi (Bronchitis) (7) (see Fig. 7.14, page 90)

Where is it? In the cavum concha, between Upper Lung and Mouth, near Oesophagus.

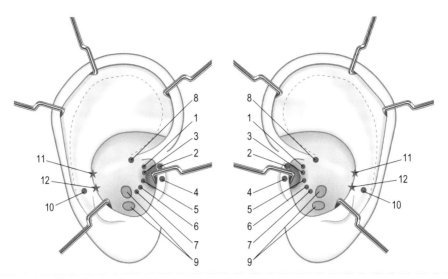

Figure 7.14 Points corresponding to the respiratory system and throat.

1. Mouth
2. Throat (C)
3. Throat (F)
4. Larynx (C)
5. Larynx (F)
6. Trachea
7. Bronchi
8. Diaphragm
9. Lung
10. Thyroid 1
11. Thyroid 2 (hormonal point)
12. Parathyroid (hormonal point)

Indications? Bronchitis, asthma, pneumonia, coughing, phlegm in the respiratory tract.

Diaphragm (8) (see Fig. 7.14)

Where is it? On the helix root, near Point Zero (it may even be the same point!)
Indications? Cramp in the diaphragm.

Lung (Pulmones, Bronchopulmonary Plexus, Bronchiectasia, Tuberculosis and Emphysema) (9) (see Fig. 7.14)

Where is it? In the cavum concha. Lung is often reckoned to be two points in each ear. In this case, Upper Lung, corresponding to the lung on the opposing side to the ear, is above Heart (C). Lower Lung, which represents the lung on the same side as the ear, lies below Heart (C). The upper part of Upper Lung coincides with the Bronchopulmonary Plexus (see page 85 under Nervous System). Lung can also be regarded as being one large zone, which covers the bottom of the cavum concha and which has Heart (C) at its centre point. In this case reckon with the right lung being reflected in the right ear and the left in the left ear. On Chinese maps there are points at the bottom edge of the lung zone called Bronchiectasia, Tuberculosis and Emphysema which may be used in cases involving these illnesses. I have chosen to describe them as a part of the Lung point.

Indications? Respiratory problems, such as asthma, coughing, pneumonia, influenza, sore throat. Nasal congestion, nasal catarrh and hoarseness are other problems which can be treated using Lung, as can addiction, to both nicotine and other drugs.

Lung can be used for pain relief and as an anaesthetic in operations (Lung is in the part of the ear innervated by the vagus nerve.)

According to TCM, the lung is one of the five large and very important yin organs, with great meaning for the lifeforce. The lungs are seen as not only as a vital part of the respiratory system but also as deciding over the whole body's qi. They are reckoned to be responsible for distributing qi and body fluids so that just enough damp and warmth reach the muscles, skin and hair. According to TCM, the lungs also regulate water passages and are responsible for the excretion of body fluids through sweat or urine. The Lung 'opens' in the nose and in the skin.

If the lung's qi is weak then, according to TCM, a series of different symptoms will occur in both body and soul. There can be breathing problems, excessive tiredness, weak voice, oedema, difficulties in urinating, and a susceptibility to catching a cold, plus shortness of breath. Also, because the lungs are responsible for distributing qi to the skin and hair, these may become dry. There may be excessive involuntary perspiration, or other deviations in the skin's proper functioning if the lungs' qi is weak. Skin troubles such as psoriasis and herpes zoster can be treated with Lung.

On the psychological plane, the lungs are linked to sorrow. If qi is weak in a person's lungs, he or she will be more susceptible to sorrow and if a person is subjected to a great deal of sorrow, this will have a debilitating effect on lung qi. However, if there is good lung qi, a person will be brave, creative, intuitive and have a keen sense of justice.

Concerning all symptoms, Lung is a good choice for treatment.

The lungs are, in addition, cleansing organs. If the body is overloaded with toxins, it is considered a good idea to treat Lung.

Lung are one of the five NADA points. In NADA acupuncture Upper Lung is treated in one ear and Lower Lung in the other.

Thyroid Gland 1 (Thyroidea, Thyroidea Plexus) (10) (see Fig. 7.14, page 90)

Where is it? Where the antihelix slopes down to the scaphoid fossa, on a level with the reflex point for cervical vertebra C1. Another thyroid gland point is sometimes drawn in the scaphoid fossa on a level with the reflex point for cervical vertebra C4. The thyroid gland also has a hormonal point, Thyroid Gland 2, see page 87.

Indications? Regulates the thyroid's functions. Used both for over- and underfunctioning.

Thyroid Gland 2, hormonal point (11) (see Fig. 7.14, page 90)

Parathyroid Gland (Parathyroidea, Endocrine Parathyroid Gland Point) (12) (see Fig. 7.14, page 90)

Where is it? On the wall of the concha, in the Zone of Control Points for the Hormonal Glands, on a level with the reflex points for cervical vertebrae C5–C6.

Indications? Dysfunctions of the parathyroid gland. Muscle cramps when the calcium metabolism is disturbed.

Tonsils (see Fig. 7.15, page 92)

Where is it? On the rear edge of the helix are several points corresponding to the tonsils. The Anatomical Atlas of Chinese Acupuncture Points (Chen 1982) gives

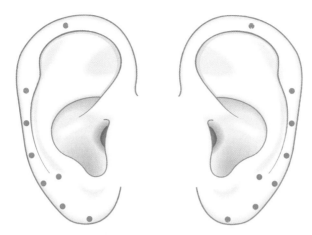

Figure 7.15 Tonsil points.

seven tonsil points on the helix. The first lies immediately behind the apex. The next lies close to LM 4, the downward edge of Darwin's tubercle. From LM 4 to the lowest part of the earlobe (LM 7) the stretch is divided into five equally long sections. Each one of these points of division contains a tonsil point. Yet another tonsil point is said to be located in the same zone as Jaw Joint.

Indications? Tonsillitis, laryngitis and other throat problems.

The intestines and the digestive system

Food is transported (see Fig. 7.16) from the mouth via the oesophagus to the stomach where it is processed. It then passes through the cardia into the small intestine (where nourishing substances are extracted) and on to the large intestine (where liquid is absorbed and the digestive process continues). When it is time for the intestine to be emptied, the excrement is moved to the rectum and emptied via the anus. The organs are represented in the ear in similar order, so too are the parts of the digestive system, reflected one after the other on the concha. The liver, gall-bladder and pancreas are other abdominal organs which play a part in the digestive process. The spleen and the thymus are organs that, among other things, play a part in the immune defence system. They will also be dealt with here.

The point Mouth is described earlier in this chapter under the heading 'The head, face and sensory organs', see page 77.

Oesophagus (2) (see Fig. 7.16, page 93)

Where is it? In the upper part of the cavum concha, between Mouth and Stomach.
Indications? Problems in the area, difficulties in swallowing, hiccup, reflux.

Upper Cardia (Cardiac Orifice, Cardia Zone) (3) (see Fig. 7.17, page 93)

Where is it? In the upper part of the cavum concha, between Oesophagus and Stomach.
Indications? Problems in the area. Gastric reflux, belching, nausea, vomiting, indigestion, heartburn, hernia.

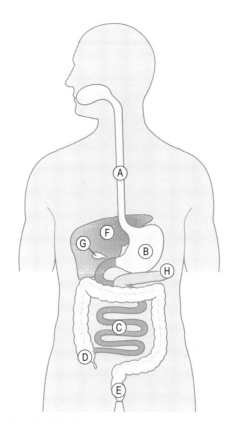

Figure 7.16

A. Oesophagus
B. Stomach
C. Small Intestine
D. Large Intestine

E. Rectum
F. Liver
G. Gallbladder
H. Pancreas

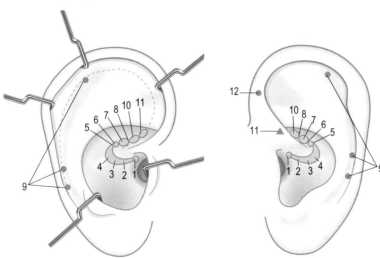

Figure 7.17 Reflex points for the intestines.

1. Mouth
2. Oesophagus
3. Upper Cardia

4. Stomach
5. Lower Cardia
6. Duodenum

7. Small Intestine
8. Appendix (F)
9. Appendix (C), three points

10. Large Intestine
11. Rectum (F)/ Haemorrhoids (F)
12. Haemorrhoids (C)

Stomach (Ventricle, Oppression Point, rear part of Solar Plexus Zone) (4) (see Fig. 7.17, page 93)

Where is it? The Stomach point lies across the helix root, near or at the centre of the concha. The zone can be larger in the left ear than in the right because the greater part of the stomach is on the left side of the body.

Indications? Stomach problems such as indigestion, heartburn, stomach ulcers. Other disturbances with digestion, such as diarrhoea, nausea, bloated abdomen. Anxiety manifested as stomach pain, anxiety before examinations, stagefright. Stomach is often used in eating disorders, both in slimming for those who eat too much and in treatment for anorexia or poor appetite. Headache and stress.

Lower Cardia (Ptosis) (5) (see Fig. 7.17, page 93)

Where is it? In the cymba concha, between Stomach and Small Intestine.

Indications? Stomach and intestinal problems or prolapse. Ptos means 'drooping organ' or 'prolapse' in Latin.

Duodenum (6) (see Fig. 7.17, page 93)

Where is it? In the lower part of the cymba concha, between Lower Cardia and Small Intestine. Sometimes Duodenum is thought to be located in the Small Intestine zone, see below.

Indications? Duodenal problems, diarrhoea, stomach rumbling, tense abdomen, irritable bowel syndrome, Crohn disease.

Small Intestine (Jejunum, Ileum, Superior Mesenteric Plexus) (7) (see Fig. 7.17, page 93)

Where is it? In the lower part of the cymba concha, between Duodenum and Large Intestine. Small Intestine is a large zone, which represents both jejunum (top part of the small intestine) and the ileum (lower part of the small intestine). If there are problems in the small intestine, there may be more than one active point in this zone. In such cases more than one point can be treated.

Indications? Problems with the small intestine, diarrhoea, stomach noises, tense abdomen, irritable bowel syndrome, Crohn disease.

According to TCM, the energy channels of the small intestine and the heart are connected. Small Intestine can thus also be used for treating problems with the heart.

Appendix (F) (Primary Appendix Point) (8) (see Fig. 7.17, page 93)

Where is it? Between Small Intestine and Large Intestine (precisely as it is in the body).

Indications? The point will be sore if the appendix is inflamed, a condition which, in the West is judged as unsuitable for treatment using ear acupuncture.

Appendix (C) (9) (see Fig. 7.17, page 93)

Where is it? Appendix (C) consists of three points, one in a finger region, one in a shoulder region and one under the Collarbone point.

Indications? The point will be sore if the appendix is inflamed, a condition which, in the West is judged as unsuitable for treatment using ear acupuncture.

Large Intestine (Colon) (10) (see Fig. 7.17, page 93)

Where is it? In the lower part of the cymba concha, near the edge of the helix, in front of Small Intestine. The large intestine is — as its name implies — a large organ and its reflex zone in the ear is also relatively large. Palpate the sore/active part of the zone. More than one active point can be found in the Large Intestine zone when there are problems with the large intestine. In such cases both can be treated.

Indications? Constipation, diarrhoea, haemorrhoids, colitis, irritable bowel syndrome, Crohn's disease. According to TCM, the energy canals for the lungs and the large intestine are connected. Large Intestine may thus be used in cases of problems otherwise treated with the Lung point, for example skin trouble.

Rectum (F) / Haemorrhoids (C) (11) (see Fig. 7.17, page 93)

Where is it? In the cymba concha, in front of Large Intestine, near Coccyx, under the edge of the helix.

Indications? Prolapse of the anus, constipation, diarrhoea, haemorrhoids, itching and cramps in the rectum, difficulties in retaining gas and faeces.

Haemorrhoids (C) (Haemorrhoidal nucleus) and Haemorrhoids (F) (12) (see Fig. 7.17, page 93)

Haemorrhoids are swellings of veins in the rectum which can bleed, itch and be painful. They may be located close to the anus and visible, or be higher up inside the rectum.

Where is it? Haemorrhoids (C) is depicted on the front edge of the helix, between the apex and the ear's upper root. Haemorrhoids (F) is depicted near Rectum (F) under the edge of the helix.

Indications? Diagnosis and treatment of external and internal haemorrhoids. Anal fissures. Rectal prolapse. Difficulties in holding gas and faeces. Pain in the anus, for example after diarrhoea.

Liver (Hepar) (1) (see Fig. 7.18, page 96)

Where is it? In the back part of the concha behind Stomach, on a level with the helix root. The reflex zone for the liver is large. Some books maintain that the Liver point is only to be found in the right ear, others that it is to be found in both ears, or that it is bigger in the right ear, though still with a smaller point in the left. Palpate the sore/active part of the zone. In the Liver Zone are points with the names Cirrhosis, Hepatitis and Hepatomegalia, (see Ch. 8, Functional points, page 120).

Indications? Problems with the liver and gallbladder.

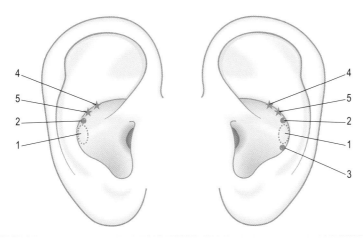

Figure 7.18 Some of the internal organs involved in digestion.

1. Liver
2. Spleen (F)/Pancreas in Left Ear. Gallbladder in Right Ear
3. Spleen (C) in Left Ear.
4. Pancreas 2 (hormonal point) (on the wall of the concha)
5. Thymus (hormonal point) (on the wall of the concha)

According to TCM, treating the point Liver can help 'stagnated liver qi' to flow smoothly. The Liver is a large and very important yin organ. In TCM the liver's function is described thus: 'The liver governs the free flow of qi and blood, harmonizes the emotions and adjusts and makes things smooth'. Because the liver's task is to see that qi and blood flow smoothly between the different organs, liver failure can be fatal. If the liver's qi stagnates, a series of different symptoms arise in both body and soul. According to TCM, stagnated liver qi can, among other things, give rise to high blood pressure, painful menstruation, poor digestion, cramps and migraine. On the psychological level, stagnated liver qi causes aggression, bad temper, frustration, stress and depression. The liver governs the efficient working of tendons and muscles and a bad function of the liver can result in stiffness, pain or other damage. In the case of all the symptoms outlined above, Liver is a good choice for treatment.

According to TCM, the liver 'opens' in the eye. This means that the Liver point can also be used to treat different eye problems, for example, dry eyes, bloodshot eyes, runny eyes and blurred vision.

The liver is also a cleansing organ whose task is to rid the body of 'toxins'. If the body is burdened with alcohol, drugs or medicines for example, it is considered a good thing to treat Liver.

Liver is one of the five NADA points. In NADA acupuncture you do not look for active points but insert needles according to a standard pattern. In such cases the needle for Liver is inserted far back in the liver's zone, right above the helix root, in both ears.

The following three organs (Gallbladder, Pancreas and Spleen) are thought by most acupuncture books to have a reflex point only in the ear on the same side as the organ. The spleen and pancreas are on the left side, under the ribcage, and the gallbladder is near the liver under the ribcage to the right. For safety's sake look for the active point in both ears!

Gallbladder (2) (see Fig. 7.18, page 96)

Where is it? In the rear part of the cymba concha in the right ear, above Liver in the zone where Spleen (F) and Pancreas are to be found in the left ear.

Indications? Problems originating in the gallbladder or pancreas, tinnitus, migraine, tendon problems.

Pancreas (Pancreatitis) (2) (see Fig. 7.18, page 96)

Where is it? Pancreas lies between Liver and Kidney (C) in the cymba concha in the left ear, in the same zone as Gallbladder in the right ear. Also to be found in the Pancreas zone is the point Pancreatitis, see Ch. 8, Functional points, page 120. The pancreas also has a hormonal point. Pancreas 2 (see page 88).

Indications? Problems with the pancreas.

Spleen (F) and Spleen (C) (Lien) (2–3) (see Fig. 7.18, page 96)

Where is it? Spleen (C) is located in the rear part of the cavum concha in the left ear below Liver. Spleen (F) is located in the rear part of the cymba concha in the left ear, above Liver in the same zone as Gallbladder in the right ear and Pancreas in the left ear.

Indications? Digestive problems, gases, gastritis, weakness in the immune system, lack of blood, muscular weakness, urinal incontinence.

According to TCM, the spleen is important for more functions than those ascribed to it in the West. The spleen in TCM is the most important organ for digestion. The spleen is responsible too for the free flow of fluids and for keeping the body's organs and fluids in place. A weak Spleen qi can, according to TCM, mean poor digestion, indigestion, heartburn, chronic diarrhoea, prolapses (such as prolapse of the uterus), varicose veins, haemorrhoids, tendency to a build-up of phlegm, weak or painful musculature, swellings, lymph and blood sickness and heavy vaginal bleeding. In of all these symptoms, Spleen is a good choice for treatment.

Pancreas 2, hormonal point (Endocrine Pancreas, Insulin Point) (4) (see Fig. 7.18, page 96)

This point is described on page 88.

Thymus, hormonal point (Thymus Gland Point, Thymic Plexus) (5) (see Fig. 7.18, page 96)

This point is described on page 88.

The heart and the circulatory system

A ground rule is that the internal organs are depicted in the concha. There are some exceptions to the rule. One example is Heart (F). The explanation for this is that the heart consists of a special sort of striated muscle and that therefore there is a depiction of it among other parts of the musculature in the reflex zone for the thorax. The heart's neurological function is to be found at the bottom of the concha and is called Heart (C).

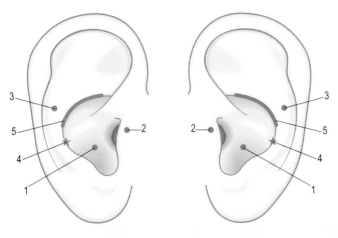

Figure 7.19 The heart and the circulatory system.

1. Heart 1 (C)
2. Heart 2 (C)
3. Heart (F)
4. Cardiac Plexus/Muscle Relaxation
5. Circulatory system

Heart 1 (C) (Cor, Vegetative Zone) and Heart 2 (C) (Cor, Vegetative Zone, Cardiac Point) (1–2) (see Fig. 7.19)

Where are they? Heart 1 (C) is in the middle of the deepest part of the concha cavum, between Upper and Lower Lung. This zone is sometimes called the Vegetative Zone and reflects not the muscular organ, the heart, but its autonomous functioning. (See too Cardiac Plexus.) Ancient Chinese texts list Heart 2 (C) in the upper part of the tragus, above Inner Ear and below External Ear.

Indications? Arrhythmias, palpitation, angina pectoris, symptoms that persist after a heart attack, high blood pressure, low blood pressure.

According to TCM, the heart has significance for, among other things, sleep, perspiration and anxiety. Heart can be treated for sleeping problems, nightmares, difficulties with concentration, anxiety, night sweat and depression. According to TCM, the heart 'opens' in the tongue. The point Heart can therefore be used to treat such problems as sores on the tongue.

Heart (F) (Cor, Vegetative Zone) (3) (see Fig. 7.19)

Where is it? On the antihelix, at a level with the cervical vertebrae.

Indications? Arrhythmias, palpitation, angina pectoris, symptoms that persist after a heart attack, high blood pressure, low blood pressure.

Cardiac Plexus (Muscle Relaxation, Middle Cervical Plexus, Middle Cervical Ganglion Point, Wonder Point, Marvellous Point, Jisong) (4) (see Fig. 7.19)

This point is described on page 86.

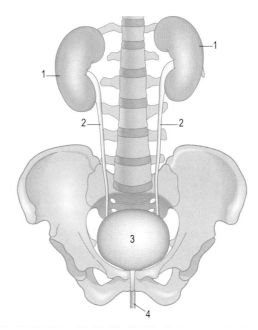

Figure 7.20 The urinary tract.

1. Kidney
2. Ureter

3. Urinary Bladder
4. Urethra

Blood and Lymph Vessels

Where are they? Blood vessels (arteries and veins) and lymph vessels are depicted in the same point as the part of the body they pass through.

Circulatory System (Blood Vessels) (5) (see Fig. 7.19, page 98)

Where is it? The zone Circulatory System is depicted on the wall of the concha, from the reflex point for cervical vertebra C7 to the reflex point for lumbar vertebra L4, in the same zone as the sympathetic trunk.

Indications? The zone represents the peripheral arteries and veins and the sympathetic nerves that regulate the blood vessels. Used to relieve symptoms of the heart's blood vessels, high blood pressure and when feet and hands are cold.

The urinary tract

The organs of the body that produce and discharge urine make up the urinary tract. The kidneys filter out liquid and waste products from the circulatory system, the ureter transports these to the urinary bladder, where it is kept until the time comes for its discharge as urine via the urethra, the last part of the tract. In men the prostate gland lies around the urethra.

The reflex zones for the urinary tract are depicted differently on the French and Chinese point maps.

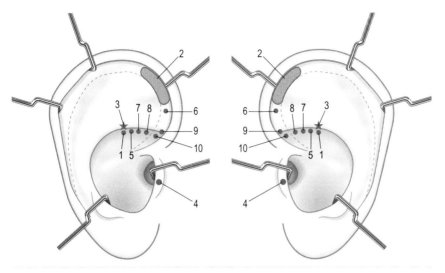

Figure 7.21 Urinary tract reflex points.

1. Kidney (C)	4. Adrenal Gland 2	8. Urethra/Prostate (C)
2. Kidney (F)	5. Ureter (C)	9. Urethra (F)
3. Adrenal Gland 1 (hormonal point)	6. Ureter (F)	10. Prostate (F)/Vagina (F)
	7. Urinary Bladder	

Kidney (C) (Renin, Angiotensin, Adrenal Gland, Cortisone) (1) and Kidney (F) (Renal Parenchymal Zone) (2) (see Fig. 7.21)

A ground rule of ear acupuncture is that the internal organs are depicted in the concha. There are some exceptions, however. One such is Kidney (F). Having developed from the mesoderm, the kidneys have a different embryological background to the other internal organs. The actual kidney organ, Kidney (F), is located under the ascending helix, part of the mesoderm. The kidney's function has a point in the concha called Kidney (C).

Where is it? Kidney (C) is in the upper part of the cymba concha, below Shen Men, above Stomach. Kidney (F) is in a zone under the helix, between the upper and lower legs of the antihelix.

Indications? Kidney and urinary troubles. Kidney (F) rather influences the organ itself than its functioning. Kidney (C) influences the kidney's function and is therefore seen to be effective in treating high blood pressure and allergies.

According to TCM, the kidneys are seen as containing the body's fundamental energy and store the vitally important essence Jing. They thus govern the process of achieving maturity and both physical and psychological development. Good kidney qi is necessary in order for reproduction and sexuality to function. The kidneys are also responsible for the skeleton, teeth and hair on the head. The kidneys are regarded as the base for yin and yang and decide a person's viability and the duration of life. According to TCM, the kidney is one of the very important, powerful yin organs.

If the kidneys' qi is weak a number of symptoms will arise in both body and soul. A person may have poor growth both physically and mentally, trouble in the urinary apparatus (for example difficulty in holding urine), impotence, backache, pains in the knees, slow healing of fractures, brittle teeth, tinnitus and poor hearing. On the psychological plane, reduced amounts of kidney qi may give rise to fear and tiredness. A person with weak kidney qi will be more easily afraid and if someone is subjected to too many fearful experiences, it will deplete kidney qi. (If a person is very scared, he or she may wet their pants.) In the case of all such symptoms the Kidney point is a good choice for treatment.

According to TCM the kidney 'opens' in the ear. This means that the Kidney point can also be used to treat ear trouble (for example impaired hearing, tinnitus and earache).

In addition, the kidney is a cleansing organ. If the body is overburdened with toxins, Kidney should be treated. Kidney (C) is one of the five NADA points (see Ch. 13, NADA: using ear acupuncture to fight addiction).

Adrenal Gland 1, hormonal point (ACTH, Glandula Suprarenalis, Cortisone) (3) (see Fig. 7.21, page 100)

This point is described on page 88.

Adrenal Gland 2 (ACTH, Cortisol, Cortisone, Glandula Suprarenalis, Skin Master Point, Anti-hypertension, High Blood Pressure) (4) (see Fig. 7.21, page 100)

The adrenal gland regulates the hormones. ACTH is short for adrenocorticotropic hormone. It is produced in the frontal lobe of the pituitary gland and governs the production of cortisol in the cortex of the adrenal gland, and thus the amount of cortisol in the body. Adrenal Gland is both a reflex point and a functional point. (On Nogier's reflex maps there is yet another point named Adrenal Gland. It covers a large zone on the ascending helix, starting just in front of Point Zero, ending at Apex.)

Where is it? On the tip of lower curve of the tragus apex, if it has two curves. In the lower part of the tragus if the tragus has one curve. Sometimes a point is indicated with the name ACTH on the inside of the tragus, subtragus, and a point with the name Cortisol is indicated a few millimetres diagonally below Adrenal Gland.

Indications? Pain, allergies and inflammation, rheumatic aches of acute or chronic character, arthrosis, skin complaints, itching, anxiety, phobias, stress, exhaustion, high blood pressure, low blood pressure.

Ureter (C) and Ureter (F) (5–6) (see Fig. 7.21, page 100)

Where are they? Ureter (C) is in the upper part of the cymba concha between Kidney (C) and Urinary Bladder (C). Ureter (F) is under the edge of the helix, below Kidney (F), on a level with the lower leg of the antihelix, near Sympathetic Autonomic Point.

Indications? Problems in the urinary tract.

Urinary Bladder (7) (see Fig. 7.21, page 100)

Where is it? Urinary Bladder is the upper part of the cymba concha between Ureter and Urethra (C), above Small Intestine.

Indications? Problems in the urinary tract, for example urinary tract infections (UTI), cystitis, enuresis, urine retention, incontinence, prostatitis.

According to TCM, pain along the urinary bladder meridian can be treated using the Urinary Bladder point. The Urinary Bladder Meridian runs over the head, then down the neck and back, through the buttocks and the back of the legs.

Urethra (C) and Urethra (F) (8–9) (see Fig. 7.21, page 100)

Where are they? Urethra (C) is in the cymba concha, between Urinary Bladder and the edge of the helix. Urethra (F) is under or on the edge of the helix, 2–4 mm below Sympathetic Autonomic Point.

Indications? Urethritis, difficulties in discharging or retaining urine, enuresis (nightly involuntary discharge of urine). Urethra is also described in Chinese texts as reflecting the prostate gland and Urethra (C) can be used in treatment of prostate trouble (for example prostatitis).

Prostate (C) and Prostate (F) (8, 10) (see Fig. 7.21, page 100)

Where are they? Prostate (C) is in the same place as Urethra (C). Prostate (F) is on the inside of the edge of the helix, in the same place as Vagina (F). (Sometimes Uterus [C] is seen as corresponding to the male Prostate.)

Indications? Prostate trouble. Urethritis and other urinary dysfunctions.

The gynaecological organs

The points relating to the sex organs are given differently on Chinese and French maps.

External Genitalia (C) (1) (see Fig. 7.22, page 103)

Where is it? External Genitalia (C) is on the ascending helix, on a level with the lower leg of the antihelix, on the outside of Sympathetic Autonomic Point.

Indications? Symptoms such as reddened skin, burning sensation, pain, itching in the external sex organ, impotence, loss of libido.

External Genitalia (F) (Sexual Desire, Bosch Point, Libido, Penis, Clitoris, E2) (2) (see Fig. 7.22, page 103)

The name Bosch sometimes given to this point derives from the 17th century Dutch artist Hieronymus Bosch's painting Garden of Lust. The painting hangs in the Prado Museum in Madrid and is full of details and symbols, among them a small black figure, skewer in hand, climbing into a human ear. One end of the skewer is in the Bosch point also known as Sexual Desire, the other in Jerome's Point, also known as Sexual Compulsion.

Where is it? External Genitalia (F) lies on the helix root where it meets the tragus, diagonally behind and below the point Weather.

Indications? Symptoms such as reddened skin, burning sensation, pain, itching in the external sex organ, impotence, loss of libido.

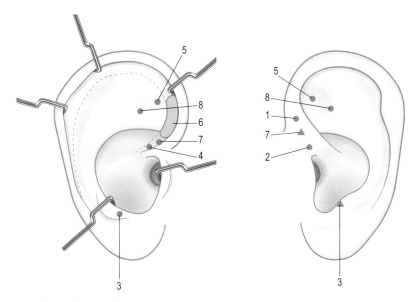

Figure 7.22 Reflex points for the gynaecological organs.

1. External Genitalia (C)
2. External Genitalia (F) / Sexual Desire
3. Ovary (C)/Testicle (C)
4. Ovary (F)/Testicle (F)
5. Uterus (C)
6. Uterus (F)
7. Vagina/Prostate (F)
8. Pelvic Girdle

Ovary (C) / Testicle (C) (Gonadotrophin, Sex Glands, Gonads, Internal Genitals) (3) (see Fig. 7.22)

Where is it? Ovary (C) is in the same point as Testicle (C), on the inside of the frontal part of the antitragus, in or close to the hormonal zone. On Chinese point maps an Ovary point is sometimes to be found close to Uterus (C).

Indications? Menstruation disturbances such as irregular or missing periods, painful periods, infertility because of poor functioning of the ovaries, menopausal problems. Sexual function disturbances, eczema on the scrotum, hormonal migraine.

Ovary (F) / Testicle (F) (Ovarium, Adnexa) (4) (see Fig. 7.22)

Where is it? Ovary (F) is in the same point as Testicle (F), on the inside of the edge of the helix, in front of Point Zero.

Indications? Menstruation disturbances such as irregular or missing periods, painful periods, infertility because of poor functioning by the ovaries, menopausal problems. Sexual function disturbances, eczema on the scrotum, hormonal migraine.

Testicle (C) (Ovary [C]) and **Testicle (F)** (Ovary [F], Ovarium, Adnexa) (3–4) (see Fig. 7.22)

Where are they? Testicle (C) is in the same point as Ovary (C), on the frontal part of the antitragus, in or close to the hormonal zone. Testicle (F) is in the same point as Ovary (F), on the inside of the edge of the helix, in front of Point Zero.

Indications? Menstruation disturbances such as irregular or missing periods, painful periods, infertility because of poor functioning by the ovaries, menopausal problems. Sexual function disturbances, eczema on the scrotum, hormonal migraine.

Uterus (C) (Womb, Tiankui, Prostata) (5) (see Fig. 7.22, page 103)

Where is it? Uterus (C) is in the fossa triangularis, about a third of the way from the edge of the helix on an imaginary line which goes from the edge of the helix to the tip of fossa triangularis, midway between the upper and lower legs of the antihelix. (Sometimes Uterus [C] is seen as corresponding to the male Prostate.) The Uterus point is sometimes depicted higher up under the edge of the helix, in the upper, forward corner of the fossa triangularis.

Indications? Various gynaecological disturbances, such as inflammation of the uterus, severe bleeding, irregular periods, discharges, pain after childbirth. Used too for disturbances in sexual function and in cases of prostatis in men. Should be used with care during pregnancy because it is thought that the point may trigger childbirth.

According to TCM, the point supports yang and gives nourishment to Jing, 'the essence', regulates menstruation and harmonises the blood.

Uterus (F) (Uterus) (6) (see Fig. 7.22, page 103)

Where is it? Uterus (F) is in a zone under the edge of the helix, starting at the level where the lower leg of the antihelix crosses the helix, close to Sympathetic Autonomic Point, and going upwards.

Indications? Various gynaecological disturbances, such as inflammation of the uterus, severe bleeding, irregular periods, discharges, pain after childbirth. Used too for disturbances in sexual function and in cases of prostatis in men. Should be used with care during pregnancy because it is thought that the point may trigger childbirth.

Vagina (Prostate [F]) (7) (see Fig. 7.22, page 103)

Where is it? On the inside of the edge of the helix, diagonally in front of/above External Genitalia (F).

Indications? Pain or other vaginal symptoms.

The Pelvic Girdle (Pelvic Bone, Hip Joint (F), Pelvic Cavity, Sacroiliac Joint) (8) (see Fig. 7.22, page 103)

Where is it? In the bottom part of the tip of the cavity of the fossa triangularis, under Shen Men.

Indications? Pelvic pain, symphysis pubis dysfunction (SPD), low back pain. Painful menstruation, pelvic-floor insufficiency, endometriosis, prostate trouble.

Chapter contents

Functional points

In this chapter we shall look at some of the ear's functional points. Functional points need not correspond to a localised part of the body but can have an influence on the entire body. Some of them are both reflex and functional points and several are important points which are used often.

Because the points have been named differently by a variety of authors, there is confusion in existing literature. In this book I have decided to employ the most commonly used names but also to give alternative terminology in parenthesis.

Balancing effect

Ear acupuncture has a balancing, homeostatic effect. The same point can be used to treat over- and under-functioning. For example, the point Hunger can be used to treat both an appetite that is too large and one that is too small. Similarly, Blood Pressure can be used to treat both high and low blood pressure.

Right or left ear?

As a rule reflex points become active in the ear on the same side as the damaged or painful body part. Functional points usually become active on the dominant side (See *Laterality* in Ch. 5, Explanatory models for acupuncture). Choose therefore in the first instance to treat functional points in the right ear of a right-handed person and in the left ear of someone who is left-handed, or treat both ears.

Masterpoints

The most powerful of the functional points are known as masterpoints.

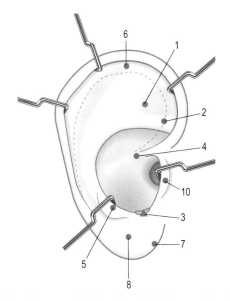
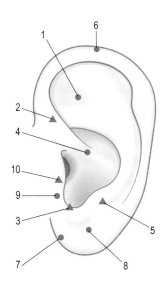

Figure 8.1 Masterpoints.

1. Shen Men
2. Sympathetic Autonomic Point
3. Endocrine
4. Point Zero
5. Thalamus
6. Allergy
7. Master Cerebral
8. Master Sensorial/Eye
9. V-point
10. Master Oscillation

Shen Men (Spirit Gate, Divine Gate) (1) (see Fig. 8.1)

Where is it? Shen Men lies in or close to (a little before and a little above) the tip of fossa triangularis which lies between the upper and lower legs of the antihelix.

Indications? Anxiety, pain, disturbed sleep, allergies.

In Chinese 'shen' means 'soul/spirit' and 'men' means 'door/gateway'. The point is sometimes called 'Heaven's gate' or 'opening to the spirit'. It is perhaps the most commonly used of all points in the ear. Some body acupuncturists use the Shen Men as a support point in all treatment. It has 'a broad spectrum of effect'. It is the most calming and relaxing ear point. It diminishes stress, pain, tension, anxiety, depression, sleeplessness, worry, impatience and oversensitivity. Shen Men also has anti-allergic and anti-inflammatory effects. It strengthens the effect of all other ear points and can therefore be used as a 'speed point' (a point which speeds up the effect of treatment on other points).

In operations where acupuncture anaesthetic is used, Shen Men is one of the most important points. It is one of the five points Oleson (1998) calls 'primary masterpoints'. Shen Men is also one of the five NADA points (NADA is a standardised form of ear acupuncture used to fight addiction; see Ch. 13).

Sympathetic Autonomic Point (Sympaticus, Autonomous Point, Vegetativum) (2) (see Fig. 8.1)

Where is it? Sympathetic Autonomic Point is both a reflex and a functional point with considerable systemic effect. It lies under the edge of the helix and is invisible when looking straight at the ear. The needle should be aligned parallel with the lower leg of the antihelix, laid under the edge of the helix and inserted at the bottom of the crease under the helix where the lower leg of the antihelix comes to an end.

Indications? Malfunctioning of the internal organs, anxiety, involuntary perspiration, night sweat, pain.

Sympathetic Autonomic Point balances the activity in both the sympathetic and parasympathetic nervous systems and is used in case of disturbances. In so doing the internal imbalance is reduced and there is a beneficial effect on various internal organs. Sympathetic Autonomic Point is thought to improve blood circulation, correct irregular and rapid heart beat and to diminish vascular spasm. Sympathetic Autonomic Point has a relaxing effect on the internal organs. Because it is antispasmodic, it is used in case of cramps, for example colic pain and problems with kidney stones and gallstones. Sympathetic Autonomic Point has a very relaxing and soothing effect in the event of stress. It is a strong painkiller and is used during acupuncture anaesthetic. According to traditional Chinese medicine (TCM), it gives nourishment to yin and supports yang.

Sympathetic Autonomic Point is one of the five points Oleson (1998) describes as 'primary masterpoints'.

It is also one of the five NADA points.

Endocrine (Hormone, Intertragus, Hypophysis, Internal Secretion, Neurohypophysis, Pituitary Gland, Anterior Pituitary, Parathoidea, Thyroidea. In the zone there are points with names like FSH, Follicle Stimulating Hormone, LH, Luteinising Hormone, ACTH [Adrenocorticotropic Hormone]), TSH [Thyroid Stimulating Hormone], Gonadotrophin, Oxytocin, Vasopressin, Prolactin) (3) (see Fig. 8.1, page 106)

Where is it? In an area comprising the inner wall of the incisura intertragica and its edge — 'in the middle of the hammock', so to speak — there are points marked on different maps with all the above names. I have chosen rather to describe it as one zone. Search for active points in this zone and use them for treatment. (The point Prolactin is in some point maps marked in the concha, closer to the external ear channel, see page 118.)

Indications? One can see the pituitary gland as the conductor of an orchestra of all the body's hormonal glands. It governs many functions via an ingenious feedback system in which the hormones act as messengers.

Endocrine point has a homeostatic effect on hormonal levels. It regulates these by lowering them if they are too high and raising them if too low. The point is thought to activate the pituitary gland, which in turn controls the other hormonal glands.

Endocrine is also used in treatment if hormone levels are unstable. Urogenital problems such as irregular menstruation, impotence, menopausal problems, infertility, amenorrhoea, retention of milk or underproduction of milk are all examples of symptoms that can be treated with Endocrine. The point may also be used for skin troubles, allergies, oversensitivity, rheumatic illnesses and inflammations because it is considered to have an anti-allergic, anti-rheumatic and anti-inflammatory effect. Do not use Endocrine on patients who are pregnant.

According to TCM, Endocrine releases stagnated liver qi, activates the blood circulation, diminishes damp and oedema.

Endocrine is one of the five points Oleson (1998) calls 'primary masterpoints'.

Point Zero (Middle Ear, Diaphragm, Ear Centre, Umbilical Cord, Hiccough, forward part of Solar Plexus Zone, Celiac Plexus) (4) (see Fig. 8.1, page 106)

Where is it? Point Zero lies on the helix root, near the crossover to the ascending helix. If you draw a screwdriver-like object (or a fingernail) along the helix root you discover a vertical notch. Point Zero is in this notch. Point Zero is nearly always active. It lies so close to Diaphragm that I have chosen to present them both here as one single point. Sometimes Diaphragm is drawn around 2 mm behind Point Zero. Solar Plexus is often drawn as a larger zone, with Point Zero in its forward section and Stomach to the rear.

(Paul Nogier describes a point, Inferior Member Master Point, that is 1 mm in front of Point Zero, and another point, Superior Member Master Point, that is also on helix's root, 3 mm in front of Point Zero. The first one has effect on the lower limbs and the second one on the arms.)

Indications? Point Zero is the centre of the ear. It corresponds to the navel or solar plexus, which are at the centre of the body. Point Zero is also an emotional centre and can calm a stressed stomach or intestine.

According to Nogier, Point Zero is also the ear's electrical centre, a 'command point' which governs the whole ear and its energy. It is thought to provide homeostasis for the whole body, to balance energy, hormonal and brain activity. Treatment of Point Zero backs up treatment of other points. It gives energy, quietens anxiety and has a relaxing effect even on muscles. Point Zero's functions are reminiscent of those of San Jiao (see page 116).

According to Chinese textbooks, Point Zero helps the energy in the stomach to travel downwards, as it should, instead of going upwards. Therefore Point Zero is good for treating nausea, vomiting and hiccups.

The general sensitivity of the ear can be influenced by Point Zero. In cases where there are no active points and thus no reflexes, treatment of Point Zero is recommended. Some experts suggest that a gold needle be used in such cases. In cases of exaggerated sensitivity, creating too many active points, treatment of Point Zero is also recommended, using a silver needle. After some minutes a new examination of the ear should be undertaken.

In his book *The Man in the Ear* (Nogier & Nogier 1985) Nogier states that Point Zero is so powerful that in many cases it is enough just to treat it. (After realizing that one of his colleagues had great problems finding the different points, Nogier decided to teach him to find just this one point, because treating it was often enough to give a positive result.)

Point Zero is the starting point for geometric ear acupuncture.[1]

Point Zero is one of what Oleson (2003) calls 'primary masterpoints'.

Thalamus (Pain Control Point, Brain, Cerebral Master Point, Dermis, Excitement) (5) (see Fig. 8.1, page 106)

Where is it? Thalamus is both a reflex point and a functional point with considerable systemic effects. It is situated low down on the inside wall of the antitragus, where the wall meets the bottom of the concha. On the inside of the antitragus

[1] In geometric acupuncture an imaginary line is drawn from Zero through an active point and the acupuncturist looks for more active points along the line. See Ch. 12, Treatment suggestions, page 171.

you'll sometimes find an indentation from the apex to the concha. Thalamus lies at the bottom of this indentation. Look for active points in the zone and treat them.

Indications? Acute and chronic pain, disturbances in the central nervous system, after stroke, and disorders in the digestive, hormonal and urogenital systems, in cases of high blood pressure, sleeping problems, sweating, swellings, anxiety and shock.

Thalamus is one of the most important of the pain-relieving points in ear acupuncture. Thalamus regulates activity in the cerebral cortex and can be used on occasions when such activity is too high or too low. According to Oleson (2003), Thalamus corresponds to the whole diencephalon, including the thalamus and hypothalamus. The Thalamus point is thought to reduce acute and chronic pain by activating the thalamus gate in the supraspinal pain inhibition system.

The point can be used to treat the types of tinnitus and bedwetting that, according to TCM, are caused by weak kidney qi. According to TCM, the kidneys are responsible for the development and efficient functioning of the central nervous system and the brain. Thalamus is also used to treat neurasthenia, exhaustion, depression and schizophrenia.

Thalamus is one of what Oleson (2003) calls 'primary masterpoints'.

Allergy (Apex, Histamine, Antihistamine) (6) (see Fig. 8.1, page 106)

Where is it? The apex is the highest point of the ear. Bend the ear forward and apply pressure so that a fold is created. Allergy lies at the top of the fold or a little further forward.

Allergy can be pricked both from below and above. If you find active points both on the underside and outside of the helix, you can choose which one to use. The point is often treated using a bleeding technique.[2]

Indications? Allergies, hay fever, asthma, poor immune defence, nettle rash. It is used also in cases of rheumatoid arthritis because it lessens inflammatory reaction. According to Chinese texts, the point can 'take away heat and wind, work as an antispasmodic, relieving pain, quietening the energy in the liver and giving clearer vision'. It is used, therefore, to treat high temperature, high blood pressure, inflamed eyes and pain.

Master Cerebral (Master Omega, Omega Head Point, Omega 0, Prefrontal Cortex, Psychotropic Zone 2, Nervosity, Neurasthenia, Worry Point, Psychosomatic 2, Anxiety Point, Bromazepam Analogue Point, Remember Point, Memory 1) (7) (see Fig. 8.1, page 106)

Where is it? On the front side of the earlobe, close to the point where the lobe meets the chin, horizontally under the level of Master Sensorial and Eye, above LM 8 and vertically in front of incisura intertragica. The point is in the zone representing the limbic system and the prefrontal lobe of the brain which is used in making decisions and starting conscious actions. There are several points in this zone whose names indicate their effect on the spiritual wellbeing.

---

[2] 'Promptly prick with three-edged needle, and let out a few drops of blood,' wrote Chen Jing (1982). Allergy has been treated like this in China for several thousand years. Read about bleeding technique in Chapter 11, Method, page 161.

Indications? Psychosomatic problems, psychological imbalance, stress, withdrawal symptoms, problems with laterality, pain, worry, all manner of anxiety, fear, fretting, poor memory, concentration problems, difficulty in taking decisions, difficulty in reassessing memories, compulsions and depression in patients with chronic pain.

Master Sensorial (Eye, Neurasthenia, Anxiety, Limbic System, Analgesic, Sensorium, Sensorial Zone) (8) (see Fig. 8.1, page 106)

Where? In the same point as Eye, in the middle of the fifth square of the earlobe. (Sometimes Master Sensorial is depicted as lying in the lobe's fourth square in front of Eye. Sensorium is considered to be located above Eye. All these points lie in the zone corresponding to the sensory part of the brain cortex.)

Indications? Anxiety, worry, sorrow, depression, poor memory, concentration difficulties, pain. Master Sensorial has a calming effect and diminishes unwelcome and exaggerated sensations from the skin, eyes and ears by influencing sensory perceptions such as sight and hearing. Master Sensorial is used to treat tinnitus and other hearing disturbances, blurred vision and other eyesight hindrances and when even mild contact is experienced as unpleasant. Sometimes used to treat vertigo and in treating addiction to alcohol and narcotics.

V-point (Valium Point, Benzodiazepine Point, Diazepam Analogue Point, Tranquilizer, Hypersensitive Point, Blood Pressure) (9) (see Fig. 8.1, page 106)

Where is it? Where the lower part of the tragus meets the cheek, halfway between LM 9 and LM 10.

Indications? The point was named when the benzodiazepine drug Valium (diazepam) was in vogue and people were more impressed by its calming effects than its harmful side effects and strong potential for addiction. Treatment of V-point can diminish anxiety, be calming and relax tense muscles. It is effective against high blood pressure, manic conditions, chronic stress, bladder irritation, insomnia, all symptoms made worse during menstruation or in menopause and when quitting smoking.

Master Oscillation Point (Laterality Point, Switching Point, Reticular System) (10) (see Fig. 8.1, page 106)

Where is it? On the subtragus, inside the tragus, level with LM 10.

Indications? 'Switching' (a point becoming active in the ear on the opposing side of the body to the particular ailment, rather than on the same side) and laterality problems. Nogier thought that people with dyslexia, learning problems, attention deficit/hyperactivity disorder (ADHD), autoimmune sicknesses, or who had a strong reaction to medicine, often suffered from problems of laterality.

Master Oscillation balances the right and left halves of the brain. It corresponds to corpus callosum, the part of the brain joining the two halves. The point is active in persons who are left-handed but mostly use their right hand, and in persons with an unclear dominance. Nogier says that when treating such patients, Master Oscillation should be stimulated before other ear acupuncture treatment is given. (Read more on laterality on pages 139 and 209.)

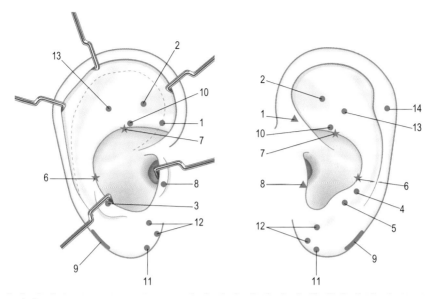

Figure 8.2 Pain relief points.

1. Sympathetic Autonomic Point
2. Shen Men
3. Thalamus
4. Neck
5. Brain
6. Muscle Relaxation
7. Adrenal Gland 1
8. Adrenal Gland 2
9. Trigeminal Zone
10. Sciatica
11. Analgesic
12. Toothache
13. Lumbago
14. Darwin's Point

Pain-relief points

Sympathetic Autonomic Point (1), Shen Men (2) and Thalamus (3), which were presented earlier in this chapter under 'Masterpoints' (see pages 105, 106 and 108), are often used as pain-relief points. Neck (4), Brain (5), Muscle Relaxation (6), Adrenal Gland 1 (7), Adrenal Gland 2 (8), Trigeminal Zone (9) and Sciatica (10) are all both reflex and functional points. They are described among the reflex points in Chapter 7, pages 74, 80, 84, 85, 86, 89 and 101. (See Fig. 8.2)

We shall now look at several other functional points whose most important use is to alleviate pain. They are used to treat many painful conditions. Some of them have other functions in addition to pain relief.

Analgesic (11) (See Fig. 8.2)

Where is it? In the seventh square on the lobe, near its forward edge, close to Prostaglandin, which is on the rear of the ear.

Indications? Severe pain, especially in the head.

Prostaglandin (see Fig. 8.3)

Where is it? On the rear of the lobe, about 2 mm from the place where the ear fastens to the cheek, near Analgesic, which is on the front of the ear. (See Fig. 8.3.)

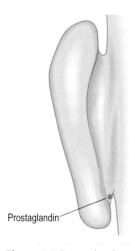

Prostaglandin

Figure 8.3 Prostaglandin.

111

Indications? Pain, particularly from inflamed joints. The point is named after a hormone-like substance prostaglandin, which is found in the body. This dilates blood vessels and has an immunodepressant effect. The point is used to treat inflammation and pain.

Toothache (Tooth Extraction, Dental Analgesia) (12) (see Fig. 8.2, page 111)

Where is it? There are several points which are used in cases of toothache and as pain relief during tooth extraction. Two of them are located in the earlobe in Squares 1 and 4 respectively. Jaw, which is in Square 3 of the lobe, can also be used in cases of toothache, along with another point in the vicinity which is located on the inside of the antitragus.

Indications? Toothache, pain relief during tooth extraction. When used to give anaesthetic if a tooth is to be extracted, electric stimulation is often needed to give adequate pain relief. The point can be treated in combination with other pain relief points.

Lumbago (High Temperature, Hot Point, Heat Point) (13) (Fig. 8.2, page 111)

Where is it? On the antihelix, where it divides into its upper and lower legs, in the Buttocks zone.

Indications? Pain in back and hips. Slight temperature with no apparent cause.

Darwin's Point (Darwin's Master Point, Bodily Defence) (14) (Fig. 8.2, page 111)

Where is it? In the groove which goes across the helix in Darwin's tubercle.

Indications? Similar effect to Shen Men when used to relieve pain. Loss of feeling and pain relief in joint problems in arms and legs, particularly pains in the lower leg.

Points that have a specific effect on psychological symptoms

In addition to Shen Men (1), Sympathetic Autonomic Point (2), Master Cerebral (3) and the V-point (4), described under the heading 'Masterpoints' (see pages 105, 106, 109 and 110), the points Neck (5), Muscle Relaxation (6) and Brain (7), described under 'Reflex points', Chapter 7, see pages 74, 80 and 86, also have a clear effect on psychological symptoms. The following points also have a clear influence on psychological symptoms such as worry, anxiety and disturbed sleep. (See Fig. 8.4, page 113.)

Jerome's Point (Sexual Compulsion, Sexual Suppression, Relaxation) (8) (see Fig. 8.4, page 113)

Where is it? In the scaphoid fossa, in the extension of a line passing through the reflex point for Cervical Vertebra C1 and Neck.

Indications? Stress, sleep disturbances, muscular tension, uncontrolled or compulsive sexuality. Diminishes sexual desire.

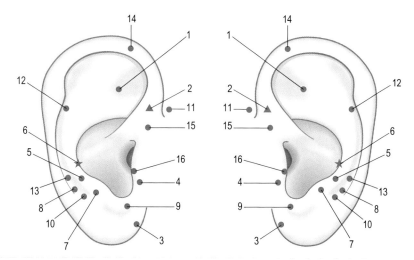

Figure 8.4 Points with particular effect on psychological symptoms.

1. Shen Men
2. Sympathetic Autonomic Point
3. Master Cerebral
4. V-point
5. Neck
6. Muscle Relaxation
7. Brain
8. Jerome's Point
9. Aggression
10. Depression
11. Psychosomatic 1
12. Insomnia 1
13. Insomnia 2
14. Omega 2
15. Frustration
16. Mania

Aggression (Irritability, Anti-aggression, Amygdala Nucleus, Lower Tragic Notch, Emotional Brain) (9) (see Fig. 8.4)

Where is it? On the lobe, 2 mm under incisura intertragica, where the cartilage ends and the lobe starts. Aggression lies in the zone corresponding to the amygdala, a part of the brain's limbic system. The amygdala regulates aggressions.

Indications? Aggression, suppressed anger, irritability, frustration, compulsive sexual actions, addiction, withdrawal symptoms.

Depression (Joy Point, Sorrow, Cheerfulness, Anti-depression, Worry) (10) (see Fig. 8.4)

Where is it? On the upper edge of the third square of the lobe, high up, where the scaphoid fossa flows into the lobe, under Neck, more or less on a horizontal level with incisura intertragica, in front of Jerome's point. Depression is situated in the same zone as Jaw Joint and Teeth.

Indications? Depression (reactive or endogenous), dejection, listlessness, sorrow, tendency to brood, menopausal problems taking the form of swings in temperament and disturbed sleep.

Psychosomatic 1 (R-point, Bourdiol Point, Psychoanalysis Point, Psychotherapy Point) (11) (see Fig. 8.4)

Where is it? A few millimetres in front of LM 1, on a level with Sympathetic Autonomic Point, where the hairline begins. It is sometimes known as the R-point after the man who discovered it, Roger Bourdiol.

Indications? Psychosomatic problems such as asthma, intestinal illnesses and skin trouble. Psychosomatic 1 is thought to influence the memory and improve cooperation between the two halves of the brain, which can make it possible to recall earlier experiences and dreams which can then be interpreted in psychotherapy.

Psychosomatic 2 (Master Cerebral) (3) (see Fig. 8.4, page 113)

There is another point named Psychosomatic 2. It is more known as Master Cerebral, see page 109.

Insomnia 1 (Wrist) (12) (see Fig. 8.4, page 113)

Where is it? In the scaphoid fossa, in or close to the Wrist point (where on the actual wrist you'll find HT 7, a cardinal point in body acupuncture treatment of sleeping problems), more or less on a level with Darwin's tubercle.
Indications? Sleeping problems, worry and depression.

Insomnia 2 (Barbiturate Analogue Point, Cushion) (13) (see Fig. 8.4, page 113)

Where is it? In the scaphoid fossa, level with LM 14, diagonally above/behind Jerome's point.
Indications? Sleeping problems, dreams.

Omega 2 (14) (see Fig. 8.4, page 113)

Where is it? On the ascending helix, above the point where the upper leg of the antihelix crosses the helix, before the apex.
Indications? Mental problems, cooperation problems, aggression, stress. Balances feelings.

Frustration (Aggression 2) (15) (see Fig. 8.4, page 113)

Where is it? In the groove between the upper edge of the tragus and the ascending helix, in front of Vitality.
Indications? Frustration, aggression, stress and addiction.

Mania (Nicotine, Hunger, Craving, Tragus Apex) (16) (see Fig. 8.4, page 113)

Where is it? On the tip of the tragus apex.
Indications? Stopping smoking, large appetite, mania (particularly concerning addiction). Traditionally used with bleeding technique (as the ear's uppermost point) to treat high temperature, inflammation, anxiety, high blood pressure, squinting, toothache and pain. (According to TCM, Tragus Apex at the top of apex's upper curve takes away heat and pain. The point at the top of the lower curve, if tragus has two curves, has the same effect in addition to being antispasmodic and taking away 'wind'.)

Addiction points

NADA treatment is a standardised form of ear acupuncture which is used in connection with counselling and social support to treat addiction to alcohol, narcotics or medicine (see Chapter 13, NADA: using ear acupuncture to fight addiction). The same five points are always used: Sympathetic Autonomic Point (1), Shen Men (2), Kidney (C) (3), Upper and Lower Lung (4–5) and Liver (6) (see Fig. 8.5). The two first named are described under Masterpoints (see pages 105 and 106), the latter three are described in Chapter 7, Reflex Points (see pages 90, 95 and 99). The NADA points are also illustrated on page 212. Listed below are several other points which influence withdrawal, craving and addiction.

Craving (Desire, Tonsil) (7) (see Fig. 8.5)

Where is it? On the back edge of the lobe, on a line between LM 14, Neck and Jerome's Point, above Metabolism. The point coincides with a Tonsil point.

Indications? Used in cases of cure from alcohol and narcotic addiction. Diminishes cravings for drugs and tobacco. Regulates appetite.

Nicotine (Hunger, Craving, Mania, Tragus Apex) (8) (see Fig. 8.5)

Where is it? On Tragus Apex if there is only one curve, or on the tip of the lower curve if tragus has two curves.

Indications? Stopping smoking, large appetite, mania (particularly concerning addiction). Traditionally used with bleeding technique (as the ear's uppermost point) to

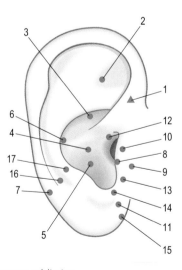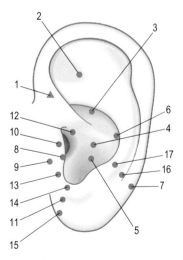

Figure 8.5 Points to treat addiction.

1. Sympathetic Autonomic Point	5. Lower Lung	10. Thirst	15. Master Cerebral
	6. Liver	11. Bridging Point	16. Jerome's Point
2. Shen Men	7. Craving	12. Mouth	17. Neck
3. Kidney (C)	8. Nicotine/Hunger/Mania	13. V-point	
4. Upper Lung	9. Hunger	14. Aggression	

treat high temperature, inflammation, anxiety, high blood pressure, squinting, tooth-ache and pain. (According to TCM, Tragus Apex at the top of apex's upper curve takes away heat and pain. The point at the top of the lower curve, if tragus has two curves, has the same effect in addition to being antispasmodic and taking away 'wind'.)

Hunger 1 and 2 (Appetite Control) (8–9) (see Fig. 8.5, page 115)

Where are they? A hunger point is situated in the grove in front of the tragus, under External Ear and External Nose (C). A second point used to regulate hunger is located on the edge of the tragus, on top of the lower curve (see 'Nicotine' above).

Indications? Regulates feelings of hunger and is used to treat both bulimia and anorexia.

Thirst (10) (see Fig. 8.5, page 115)

Where is it? In the groove in front of the upper half of the tragus, near the tip of the apex, if the apex is on a curve.

Indications? Increased thirst, dry mouth.

Bridging Point (11) (see Fig. 8.5, page 115)

Where is it? Bahr shows a point which he calls the Bridging Point on the lobe, between Aggression and Master Omega.

Indications? Addiction.

Other points often used in addiction are Mouth (12) (see page 77), V-point (13) (see page 110), Aggression (14) (see page 113), Master cerebral (15) (see page 109), Jerome's point (16) (see page 112) and Neck (17) (see page 74).

More functional points

Some of the functional points listed below are also reflex points. Hypothalamus (1), Solar Plexus (2), Vagus nerve 1 and 2 (3–4) and Thymus (5) (see Fig. 8.6, page 117) have a comprehensive effect and are described in Chapter 7, on pages 81, 83, 84 and 88.

San Jiao (Triple Heater, Triple Burner, Triple Warmer, Triple Energiser) (6) (see Fig. 8.6, page 117)

San Jiao is a concept that is to be found only in China. It describes more a function than an organ. San Jiao means 'the three burners'. The topmost burner corresponds to the organs in the thorax, above the diaphragm, which is to say those concerned with breathing. The middle burner corresponds to the organs in the region above the stomach, that is those concerned with digestion. The lower burner corresponds to the organs lower down in the abdomen, those belonging to the urogenital and gynaecological systems. If San Jiao is functioning well all these organs work well together. San Jiao is also considered to be important in the process that allows optimal transportation of fluids in the body.

Where is it? In the cavum concha, below Vagus Nerve (which is thought to have a similar function).

Indications? Disturbances in the internal organs. Problems in the breathing and digestive organs, the urinary tract and the gynaecological organs.

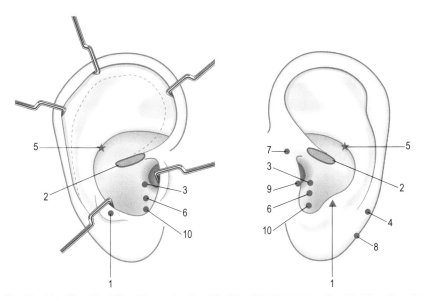

Figure 8.6 More functional points.

1. Hypothalamus
2. Solar Plexus
3. Vagus Nerve 1
4. Vagus Nerve 2
5. Thymus
6. San Jiao
7. Vitality
8. Metabolism
9. Tragus Apex
10. Prolactin

According to TCM, San Jiao helps the body to transport fluids so that they do not build up. It is also thought to take away itching and heat and is used to treat swellings, chronic constipation and problems with organs in the ribcage and abdomen.

Laterality (Tragus Master Point)

Where is it? About 3 cm in front of the ear on a level with the tragus apex. (Really this is no ear acupuncture point because it is situated on the cheek in front of the ear.)

Indications? Disturbance in laterality. Powerful pain alleviation effect. According to Paul Nogier: 'Tonus and control, external genital organs. '

Vitality (Interferon) (7) (see Fig. 8.6)

Where is it? A few millimetres under the point where the upper part of the tragus meets the antihelix, behind Frustration.

Indications? A tendency to infections, protracted infections, recovery following immune sickness, AIDS, cancer. The point is anti-inflammatory and increases immune defences.

Metabolism (Masterpoint for Metabolism) (8) (see Fig. 8.6)

Where is it? In the sixth square of the lobe, below Craving.

Indications? Problems with digestion, metabolic illnesses. A tendency to brood. It is also a tonsil point.

According to TCM metabolism is connected to the spleen. In the Nordic countries a tendency to melancholic brooding is traditionally blamed on the spleen. A popular Swedish synonym for 'melancholy' is 'mjältsjuka' ('spleen sickness').

Tragus Apex (Hunger, Mania, Nicotine) (9) (see Fig. 8.6, page 117)

Where is it? Tragus Apex is the part that protrudes most on the tragus. The tragus is sometimes divided into an upper and a lower curve. In this case Tragus Apex lies at the top of the upper curve. The points Hunger, Thirst, Mania and Nicotine are also to be found at Tragus Apex.

Indications? Stopping smoking, large appetite, mania (particularly concerning addiction). Regulates feelings of hunger and is used to treat both bulimia and anorexia. Traditionally used with bleeding technique (as the ear's uppermost point) to treat high temperature, inflammation, anxiety, high blood pressure, squinting, toothache and pain.

(According to TCM, Tragus Apex at the top of the upper curve takes away heat and pain. The point at the top of the lower curve, Lower Tragus Apex, has the same effect in addition to being antispasmodic and removing 'wind'.)

Prolactin (LTH) (10) (see Fig. 8.6, page 117)

Where is it? Most hormonal points are clustered close to the incisura intertragica, and the acupuncturist searches for active points in this zone when there are hormonal problems. A point named Prolactin is in some point maps marked a bit higher up in the concha, closer to the under ear channel.

Indications? Problems with breastfeeding, underproduction of milk.

Liver Yang 1 (1) (see Fig. 8.7, page 119)

Where is it? On the upper line of division of Darwin's tubercle, near LM 3.

Indications? Hepatitis and other disturbances in the liver. According to TCM, the point is used when there is 'liver qi stagnation' and on occasions when 'liver yang rises'.

Liver Yang 2 (Liveliness, Alertness) (2) (see Fig. 8.7, page 119)

Where is it? On the lower line of division of Darwin's tubercle, close to LM 4.

Indications? Hepatitis, other liver disturbances. According to TCM the point is used in cases of 'liver qi stagnation' and on occasions when 'liver yang rises'. Treatment of the point is thought to make the patient more lively and alert.

Omega 1 (Hypogastric Plexus, Inferior Mesenteric Ganglion, Lumbosacral Splanchnic Nerve, Mercury Toxicity, E1) Can be found described under the name Hypogastric Plexus in Ch. 7, Reflex points. (3) (see Fig. 8.7, page 119)

Where is it? In the cymba concha, beneath and slightly inclined, in front of the Urinary Bladder and between it and Small Intestine/Large Intestine on a level with Weather and External Genitalia (F).

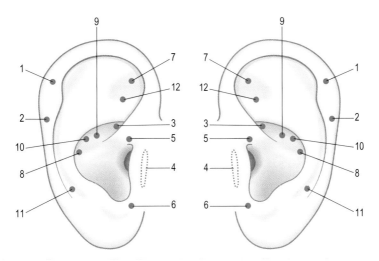

Figure 8.7 More functional points.

1. Liver Yang 1
2. Liver Yang 2
3. E1/Omega 1
4. Omega Prim
5. E2/Sexual Desire
6. E3/ Pineal Gland
7. Hepatitis 1
8. Cirrhosis/Hepatitis 2
9. Ascites
10. Pancreatitis
11. Nephritis
12. Constipation

Indications? Influences the autonomous nervous system. Used when there are problems urinating or with the functioning of the intestines. Overload of amalgam, and other environmental factors.

Omega Prim (4) (see Fig. 8.7)

Where is it? Omega Prim (or O') can move upwards or downwards in the vertical groove that is situated in front of the tragus. There is always a point that can be registered in this groove. It represents the corpus callosum, which links the right and left halves of the brain.

Indications? Omega Prim is used in cases of laterality disturbance and if the patient has psychological problems.

E Points (3, 5, 6) (see Fig. 8.7)

In addition to Master Oscillation Point and Omega Prim, described earlier in this chapter, the following points are also thought to be significant in cases of laterality disturbance.

According to Nogier, there are three E points, E1, E2 and E3. 'E' stands for 'Epiphys', the Latin term for Pineal Gland, synonymous with corpus pineale, an appendage of the upper brain. It is a hormonal gland which secretes melatonin. The E points are also known as adaptation and second points.

Where are they? E1 is in the cymba concha (See Omega 1, Hypogastric Plexus, page 84), E2 is situated where the upper part of the tragus meets the ascending helix (See External Genitalia (F)/Sexual Desire, page 122) and E3 is under the intertragic notch (see Pineal Gland, page 82).

Indications? According to Nogier, they should be treated first, before other treatment of the ear, if they are active. They are active in cases of laterality disturbance and should be treated with regular acupuncture needles very quickly – in a second – hence the alternative terminology: second points.

Hepatitis 1 and Hepatitis 2 (7–8) (see Fig. 8.7, page 119)

Where are they? There are two points called Hepatitis. The first, Hepatitis 1, is located in fossa triangularis, between Asthma and Shen Men. The second, Hepatitis 2, is in the cavum concha, in the Liver Zone.
Indications? Hepatitis, cholecystitis.

Cirrhosis (Hepatomegalia, Hepatitis 2) (8) (see Fig. 8.7, page 119)

Where is it? In the lower part of the Liver Zone, behind Stomach.
Indications? Cirrhosis of the liver, enlarged liver, hepatitis.

Ascites (Biliary Point, Alcoholism, Alcoholic Point, Drunk Point) (9) (see Fig. 8.7, page 119)

Where is it? In the cymba concha, between Kidney (C), Pancreas and Small Intestine.
Indications? Cirrhosis of the liver, ascites (a condition in which fluid collects in the abdomen because of poor functioning of the liver), alcoholism and hangover.

Pancreatitis (10) (see Fig. 8.7, page 119)

Where is it? In the cymba concha, near or in the point Pancreas.
Indications? Pancreatitis (inflammation of the pancreas), problems with digestion, migraine.

Nephritis (11) (see Fig. 8.7, page 119)

Where is it? On the border between the tail of the helix and the scaphoid fossa, on a level with LM 9.
Indications? Nephritis (inflammation of the kidney).

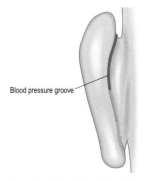

Constipation (12) (see Fig. 8.7, page 119)

Where is it? In the lower part of the fossa triangularis, parallel with the lumbar vertebrae.
Indications? Constipation.

Blood pressure groove

Blood Pressure Groove

Where is it? The groove on the rear of the ear (see Fig. 8.8 beside (3)).
Indications? High blood pressure. Chinese texts recommend bleeding technique.

Figure 8.8 Blood Pressure Groove.

Blood Pressure (High Blood Pressure, Hypertension, Depressing Point, Lowering Blood Pressure Point, Blood Pressure Control, Anti-hypertension, Renin/Angiotensin Point) (1) (see Fig. 8.9, page 122)

Where is it? The Blood Pressure point is in the upper part of the fossa triangularis, closer to the edge of the helix than the tip of the fossa triangularis, near the zone for Toes. Sometimes the point is drawn in under the edge of the helix.

Indications? Regulates blood pressure. Gives relaxation.

According to TCM, Blood Pressure calms the liver and removes wind.

Low Blood Pressure (Hypotension, Rising Pressure) (2) (see Fig. 8.9, page 122)

Where is it? Between Eye 1 and Eye 2, near the hormonal zone, a few millimetres below LM 9.

Indications? Low blood pressure. (It is likely that this point also regulates blood pressure.)

Beta-1 Receptor Point (Beta Blocker Point) and Beta-2 Receptor Point (Beta Mimetic Point) (3–4) (see Fig. 8.9, page 122)

Where are they? These two points are in the scaphoid fossa, half hidden under the edge of the helix, on a level with the lower leg of the antihelix, a few millimetres from one another.

Indications? Beta-1 Receptor Point is used in cases of high blood pressure. Beta-2 Receptor Point is used to treat asthma.

Asthma 1 (Antihistamine, Dysphnea, Ding Chuan, Ping Chuan) (5) (see Fig. 8.9, page 122)

Where is it? In the upper part of the fossa triangularis, near, or right above Knee (C).

Indications? Asthma, bronchitis, shortness of breath, coughing, allergies, itching.

Asthma 2 (Ding Chuan, Ping Chuan) (6) (see Fig. 8.9, page 122)

Where is it? On the top of the antitragus.

Indications? Asthma, bronchitis, shortness of breath, coughing, allergies, itching.

Bronchitis (7) (see Fig. 8.9, page 122)

Where is it? In the cavum concha, between the Upper Lung point and Mouth, in the Bronchial Zone.

Indications? Bronchitis, asthma, pneumonia, coughing, phlegm in the breathing tracts.

Cough (Cough Relieving Point) (8) (see Fig. 8.9, page 122)

Where is it? On the antitragus, near Brainstem and Dizziness (perhaps it is the same point?).

Indications? Coughing.

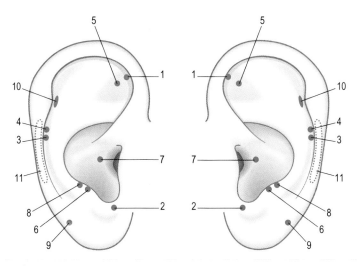

Figure 8.9 More functional points.

1. Blood Pressure	4. Beta-2 Receptor Point	7. Bronchitis	10. Urticaria Groove
2. Low Blood Pressure	5. Asthma 1	8. Cough	11. Skin Disorder
3. Beta-1 Receptor Point	6. Asthma 2	9. Sneezing	

Sneezing (9) (see Fig. 8.9)

Where is it? In the sixth square of the lobe, near the Trigeminal Zone.
Indications? Frequent sneezing caused by allergy.

Urticaria Groove (Nettle Rash, Interior Tubercle, Urticaria Point, Skin Disorder [C], Allergy Point, ACTH) (10) (see Fig. 8.9)

Where is it? In the scaphoid fossa, near Wrist, on a level with Darwin's tubercle. (On the actual wrist the body acupuncture point LU 9 is located. LU 9 is a cardinal point in treating skin disorders.)
Indications? Allergy, rash, eczema and itching. According to TCM, it takes away wind.

Skin Disorder (11) (see Fig. 8.9)

Where is it? In a long zone on the descending part of the helix. The zone starts under Darwin's tubercle and continues downwards until it is level with C1.
Indications? Rash, eczema and itching.

Sexual Desire (External Genitalia [F], Bosch Point, Sexual Desire, Libido, Penis, Clitoris, E2) (1) (see Fig. 8.10, page 123)

The name Bosch sometimes given to this point derives from the 17th century Dutch artist Hieronymus Bosch's painting Garden of Lust. The painting hangs

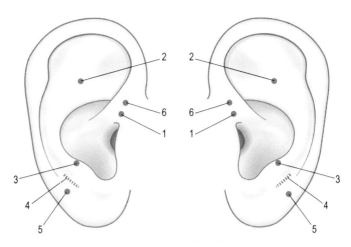

Figure 8.10 More functional points.

1. Sexual Desire
2. High Temperature
3. Dizziness
4. Auditory Zone
5. Tics
6. Weather

in the Prado Museum in Madrid and is full of details and erotic symbols, among them a small black figure, skewer in hand, climbing in an outer ear. One end of the skewer is in the point known as Sexual Desire, the other in Jerome's Point, Sexual Compulsion.

Where is it? Sexual Desire lies on the helix root where it meets the tragus, diagonally behind and below the point Weather.

Indications? Symptoms such as reddened skin, burning sensation, itching in the external sex organ, impotence, loss of libido.

High Temperature (Lumbago, Hot Point, Heat Point) (2) (see Fig. 8.10)

Where is it? On the antihelix, where it divides into its upper and lower legs, in the Buttocks zone.

Indications? A slight temperature for no apparent reason. Pains in back and hips.

Dizziness (Vertigo) (3) (see Fig. 8.10)

Where is it? On the antitragus, near Brainstem and Cough (perhaps it is the same point?).

Indications? Dizziness.

Auditory Zone (Auditory Line, Acoustic Line, Temporal Cortex, Temporal Lobe) (4) (see Fig. 8.10)

Where is it? On the earlobe, as a horizontal elongated zone in the extension of the scaphoid fossa, below the antitragus.

Indications? Impaired hearing, tinnitus, Ménière's disease.

Tics (Blepharospasmus) (5) (see Fig. 8.10, page 123)

Where is it? In the third square of the lobe, behind Tongue.

Indications? Tics (involuntary muscle contractions) in the eye. (Blepharospasmus is Latin for tics in the eye.)

Weather (6) (see Fig. 8.10, page 123)

Where is it? On the ascending part of the helix, in front of and above Outer Genitalia (F).

Indications? Symptoms which can be accentuated by a change in the weather, for example headaches, sleeping problems, pain.

Equipment

We shall now look at the 'tools' normally used in ear acupuncture.

Mechanical point detectors: probes

The simplest way of finding sore points in the ear is to palpate the ear with a mechanical point detector. Such a probe has a tip at one end so thin it can give distinct pressure on a very small surface, yet so blunt that it doesn't hurt. This tip can be fixed (without a spring) or spring-loaded. The spring-loaded part of the probe may be graduated so you can see how hard you are pushing. This makes it easier to apply equal pressure when looking for active points. The probe is usually made of metal. A thicker glass rod is used when certain points in the ear need to be massaged.

A probe can also be a great help when you are attaching pellets or seeds.

On some probes the other end is flat like a screwdriver or looks like a stirrup. The 'screwdriver' or 'stirrup' is drawn slowly along raised structures such as the antihelix or helix root and makes it easier to locate sore points or landmark grooves in such parts of the ear. (See Figs 9.1 and 9.2.)

Electrical point detectors

To find active points more easily and exactly, an electrical point detector can be used. This is an instrument that measures the skin's electrical resistance. In active points the electrical resistance will be either lower or higher than in the surrounding tissue.

There are different types of electrical point detectors. On contact with an active point an indicator bulb will light. Some point detectors also emit a sound signal. Electrical point detectors should be calibrated to take account of the sensitivity of each patient. If this is too high, more points will register than are worth treating, if too low, points may be missed. Some instruments have a calibration based on resistance at Point Zero, which is always electrically active, others based on resistance on the lobe. Read the instructions for the instrument you are using.

The probes on advanced point detector are in two parts, a probe and its sheath, both of them spring-loaded.

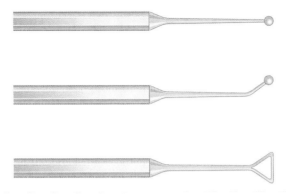

Figure 9.1 Probes, one straight and one curved with ball-tips, and one with stirrup-shaped tip.

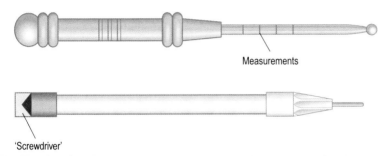

Measurements

'Screwdriver'

Figure 9.2 Two spring-loaded probes, one with graduated scale and one with screwdriver-shaped tip.

The instrument measures voltage differences between the points that the inner probe makes contact with and the surroundings touched by the sheath. In addition to finding active points, such an instrument will also tell you if the electrical resistance in the point is higher or lower than in the surrounding tissue (yellow or green bulbs light up) (see Figs 9.3 and 9.4). Such information can be of value in more specialised types of treatment. When it comes to regular ear acupuncture, with which we are concerned here, the patient is treated in the same way whether skin resistance is high or low.

With an instrument of this type, in addition to looking for active points, you can also give treatment by using the probe to send an electrical impulse through the point. Such treatment can be an alternative to acupuncture in dealing with patients who are afraid of needles.

Thus, the advantage of an advanced point detector is that it can provide information and also be used for treatment. The disadvantage is that it is more difficult to calibrate, clean and handle. The patient has to hold a probe and a wire goes from the probe to a battery-driven box. Another wire goes from the box to the probe of the instrument, held by the operator.

There is a simplified variant of an electrical point detector that resembles a thick metal pen (see Fig. 9.5). It has no wires and the patient doesn't have to hold a probe. On the other hand the acupuncturist must touch the patient with one hand while calibrating the instrument and making the initial examination. The easiest way is to hold the ear with the hand that is not holding the instrument. The pen can be

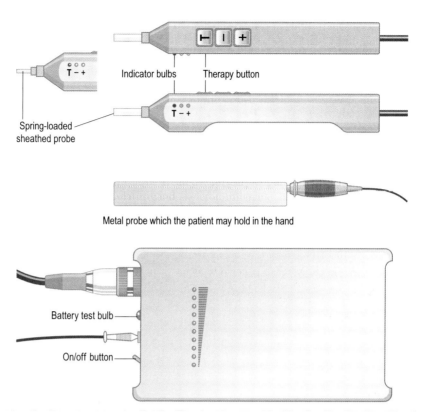

Indicator bulbs Therapy button

Spring-loaded
sheathed probe

Metal probe which the patient may hold in the hand

Battery test bulb

On/off button

Figures 9.3 and 9.4 Advanced electrical point detector. The spring-loaded probe is in two parts, probe and sheath.

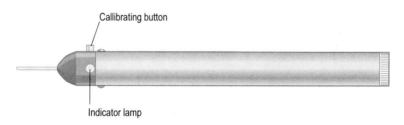

Callibrating button

Indicator lamp

Figure 9.5 Simple electrical point detector.

calibrated in a second by simultaneously holding the tip to the ear lobe and pressing a button. Then the tip is drawn across the skin with a light, even pressure. The tip must be held at the right angle — only the tip should make contact with the ear.

The most usual error made in using this simple point detector is that the acupuncturist lets go of the patient's ear (at which point the pen ceases to work) or that a protruding part of the ear involuntarily touches part of the probe (in which case the pen gives a false reading). The disadvantage with this simple point detector compared with the more advanced models is that you can't stimulate the point with electrical impulses. The advantage is that it is easy to calibrate and keep clean, considerably cheaper and can be kept in your pocket, greatly increasing the likelihood of its being used.

The various types of acupuncture needles

There are traditional acupuncture needles that stay in the ear for 30–45 minutes and then are taken out. I choose to call these 'regular' needles. In ear acupuncture semi-permanent needles are also used. These can stay in place for several days.

Sterile disposable needles

In the old days acupuncturists used needles that were sterilised between treatments and could be used again. If the sterilisation wasn't handled properly viruses such as hepatitis could survive and spread among patients. Now both national authorities and acupuncture associations insist that disposable needles be used. Blood collection agencies such as the American Red Cross or Britain's National Blood Service refuse donors who have been given recent acupuncture unless they can produce evidence that the acupuncture needles were only used once.

The acupuncture needle should be sterile until insertion. You'll find an expiry date on every box. Make sure too that packaging is unbroken so that the needles are sterile. Always wash your hands before you start treatment and be careful not to touch the tips of needles.

A needle that has been inserted in the skin but fallen out should be replaced with a new, clean one. (If you use packs of needles then make sure you use all the needles in the pack within four hours once the seal is broken.)

Used needles are regarded as dangerous waste (they are both sharp and can hold contagious matter) and should be put immediately into a special container for dangerous waste. You can't know which of your patients may be the carrier of an infectious disease. Always consider the fact that each needle, each cotton bud or dressing used to stem bleeding could be infected. Your local authority will most likely run a special service collecting dangerous waste. Check with them before you start, unless you are working in a hospital or clinic where such a service is already in operation.

Regular acupuncture needles

A regular acupuncture needle comprises a needle tip, body and handle, which can be made of different materials. Acupuncture needles can be of different lengths and thicknesses, sometimes coated with silicone. The needles may be packed with or without a protective tube or a guide tube, be packed individually or in bunches of five, 10 or 20 and be of different degrees of sharpness. The type of needle or packaging you use is a matter of personal choice and can depend on price.

Different types of needles

In traditional Chinese medicine (TCM) it is thought that, in addition to the choice of point, the material the needle is made of and the needle technique may also contribute to the effect. Acupuncture needles can be manufactured of stainless steel, gold or silver.

The most common needles are made of surgical steel (a sort of stainless steel). Their effect, according to TCM, is neutral, normalising. They contain, like other products made of surgical steel (for example, cannulae, sampling needles and scalpels) a small amount of nickel. Despite the fact that gold-plated needles are much more expensive than those of steel, they may sometimes be used on patients who are hypersensitive to nickel. Another alternative for patients who have an allergy to nickel is to treat the point electrically (see Electrical point detectors) or to use low-allergy-risk pellets (see below, pages 132–133). Seeds also contain no metal.

Some acupuncturists claim that different metals have a different effect on the body. In TCM gold needles are considered to have a reinforcing and strengthening effect and to concentrate energy, while silver needles are seen to be reducing, dispersing, draining, thus spreading energy. Nogier thought that because gold and silver have different electrical potentials the body's cells react differently to needles made from these metals. The needles generate different microstreams of electricity and the influence of these ions can affect cell information. He compared the effect of the metal to that of a valve regulating the flow of liquid through a pipe. 'An acupuncture needle cannot take away or add to an ounce of energy. Its function is to steer this energy through the body in order to distribute it in better fashion to the organs' he wrote in *The Man in the Ear* (Nogier & Nogier 1985).

The handle of the needle can also be made of various materials. Needles with spring type copper handles are common. The handle can also be made of the same material as the body of the needle, most often surgical steel, or be made of plastic. If the latter is the case, electricity cannot be used.

Japanese acupuncture needles are often coated with silicon. They slip easily through the tissue and their insertion is almost pain free. (In Japanese acupuncture the de qi effect is not sought after as it is in Chinese acupuncture.) In ear acupuncture there is no reason to use silicon-coated needles. The needle is inserted only 2–3 mm and if the ear acupuncturist has a good needle technique the insertion should not be experienced as painful.

What size of needle is suitable?

There are needles of different length and diameter. The length of a needle does not usually include its handle. In body acupuncture needles that are up to 125 mm in length are used. For ear acupuncture a suitable length is 13–15 mm. If a longer needle is used, the centre of gravity will be located further out, and the needle can more easily fall out or be pulled out inadvertently if the patient has long hair. A shorter needle (5–7 mm needles are manufactured and used, for example, in cosmetic acupuncture) is difficult to guide in the ear and demands greater agility with the fingers.

The thinnest acupuncture needles are 0.12 mm. Needles up to 0.9 mm in diameter are manufactured but needles thicker than 0.3 mm are seldom used clinically. An ear acupuncture needle should be 0.20–0.25 mm in diameter. A thicker needle will be more likely to be felt by the patient. (Some authors claim that a thicker needle can be better for certain methods of treatment if the acupuncturist wants to exert stronger stimulation of the point, or to cause bleeding.)

Packaging of needles

Acupuncture needles are packed under sterile conditions in plastic packs with a backing of paper or metal foil. In my experience, most acupuncturists find packs backed with paper quicker and easier to work with than those backed with foil.

The needles can be individually packed or in batches of five, 10 or 20. If you are working in NADA acupuncture (in which five needles are inserted into each ear) then obviously, packs of five or ten are extremely practical. However, even many other acupuncturists prefer to buy their needles in packs of five, 10 and 20. This saves time, means less packaging to be dealt with, less storage space taken up, is

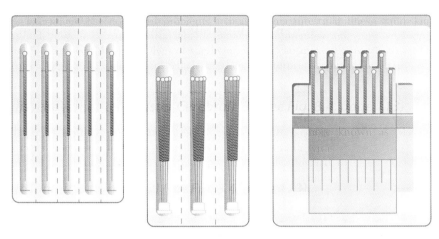

Figure 9.6 Individually packed needles, needles in batches of five and a variant of the 10-pack (EZY-10).

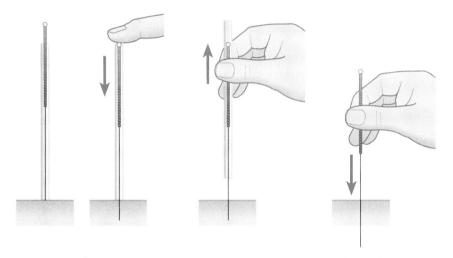

Figure 9.7 The acupuncturist can use a tube as an aid to inserting the needle.

better for the environment and more economic (needles bought in batches usually come cheaper). (See Fig. 9.6.)

With or without tube

Sometimes acupuncture needles are individually packed in a plastic guide tube. The tube is a few millimetres shorter than the needle. When the tube is held against the skin, the handle of the needle will protrude a few millimetres from the tube. With one quick thrust, the acupuncturist pushes down the needle, lifts off the tube and then carefully continues to insert the needle to the required depth (see Fig. 9.7). This can be a great help in body acupuncture when longer needles are used. In ear acupuncture when the needle is inserted just 2–3 mm, most acupuncturists use needles

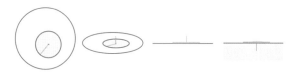

Figure 9.8 Press tacks.

without tubes. (The tubes described here are different from those used when needles are packed in batches of five. There the task of the tube is to keep the needles together.)

Semi-permanent needles

A semi-permanent needle is small and can stay in the ear for up to 10 days. For reasons of hygiene the needle should then be taken out, if it hasn't already fallen out of its own accord.

A semi-permanent needle has advantages for the acupuncturist because it is easily and quickly put in place and advantages too for the patient, who will not need as many treatments. The stimulation from semi-permanent needles is continuous, as long as the needle is in place.

There are different types of semi-permanent needles. The most common are press tacks and ASP-type needles.

Press tacks

Press tacks are also known as ear tacks, press needles or studs. They look like small drawing pins (see Fig. 9.8), are fastened to a small band aid and are often put in place with a pair of tweezers. They come in two sizes; 1.5-mm tacks are used where the ear is tougher to penetrate and 1.8-mm tacks in softer sections such as the lobe.

Press tacks too must be sterile. Some manufacturers deliver them in large packages. Be sure to choose a package in which the tacks are packed separately so you don't have to jettison the rest of the packet simply because you have opened it for one tack.

The advantage of press tacks compared with ASP-type needles is that they are considerably cheaper and, because they are thinner, they cause less pain on insertion.

ASP-type needles

A second type of semi-permanent needle is the ASP, or Aiguilles Semi-Permanentes needle (ASP is the original, manufactured in France since 1978, but other brands are now also available. See Fig. 9.9) Such needles are made in nickel-free steel, gold plate and titanium (the most biocompatible metal). ASP needles are packed in a plastic tube which is divided in the middle. If the tip of the tube is held over the chosen point in the ear with light pressure, one part of the tube slides into the other and the needle is propelled into the skin with a characteristic click. The ASP needle is in the form of a spool, which facilitates its staying in place. The needle can be covered with a small band aid.

At the other end of the tube there's a magnet. The patient can take the tube home and now and again stimulate the needle with the magnet for a stronger effect.

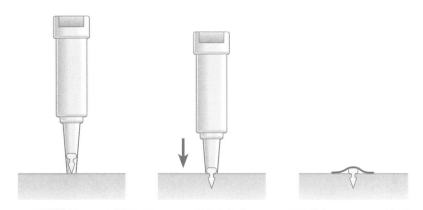

Figure 9.9 ASP-type needle.

Figure 9.10 Pellets and seeds create an indentation in the ear.

The advantage of the ASP needle compared to the press tack is that it is easier to insert exactly where you want it and that, thanks to the spool formation, it will not easily slip out.

Pellets and seeds

Instead of treating a point in the ear by inserting a needle, you can tape a pellet to the point (see Fig. 9.10). This is a little ball, or a seed, which is fastened to the point with a small band aid. The ball exerts a continual pressure on the acupuncture point. Technically speaking, because no needle is inserted in the skin, such treatment is not acupuncture but rather a form of acupressure. While pellets are rarely used in body acupuncture, they are often used in the ear (they are also used on the hands and the feet in Su Jok; see Ch. 4, Other microsystems). Pellets are an asset in the case of patients with a fear of needles, children and patients who, for diverse practical reasons, can't be treated as often as might be desirable.

Organic seeds and gold, silver and magnetic pellets

Practitioners of TCM believe that it is not just choices of point and stimulation technique that are important but also the choice of material. Pellets come in different materials, usually — like most acupucture needles — in stainless steel; but they may also be gold- or silver-plated. In TCM steel is seen as neutral. Gold pellets are considered to have a reinforcing and strengthening effect and to concentrate energy, while silver ones are thought to be reducing and dispersing. There are also magnetic pellets and gilded magnets as well as band aids containing organic seeds. Mustard and vaccaria seeds are commonly used.

As with other items made of surgical steel, steel pellets contain a small amount of nickel. If the patient experiences a reaction to the metal, the plaster must be removed and the skin allowed to rest until it is healed. Then you can try with pellets of another type. There are pellets made of allergy-proof platinum and gold-plated pellets, or you can try organic seeds.

If sensitive patients react to the band aid encasing the pellet, try another make.

Ear acupuncturists who are good with their hands and on a low budget make their own pellets. They use a small plastic or wooden plate with indentations to accommodate the seeds or pellets. A wide plaster is then taped over them and trimmed with a razor blade until they are the right size.

Transcutaneous electrical stimulation

Acupuncturists who want to combine the insertion of needles with electrical stimulation may use a transcutaneous electrical nerve stimulation (TENS) unit. This can be either battery or mains operated. The principle of TENS is that it transmits a weak stream of electricity into the body via electrodes fastened to the area causing pain, it being used primarily on the body, for pain relief. When used in acupuncture, the current is transmitted via small crocodile clips into regular needles inserted in acupuncture points. Such electrical stimulation of acupuncture needles is known as electroacupuncture (EA).

The electrodes used for TENS treatment of the body is far too large to be used in the ear. However, there is a unit like TENS in mini-format called AcuStim which has very small silver paper electrodes and this is used in the ears. When treating a patient with AcuStim, these tiny electrodes are glued to the chosen points in the ear, small-diameter cables are then used to connect them to the battery driven unit and patients can themselves turn the unit off and on, according to their needs. It can be used in treating pain or as an aid to slimming.

Moxa

The burning of moxa, a herb often used in Chinese medicine, is a natural part of acupuncture as it is practised in China (see Ch. 2, A brief look at traditional Chinese medicine). Moxa warms the body and is thought to reinforce and spread qi. It is used less often in the West.

Moxa is sold loose or in sticks that resemble cigars. It can be of various qualities, from the simpler sort to that which is specially picked and treated, and that is of course more expensive.

If loose-weight moxa is used in body acupuncture, it is usually burned in a moxa box, made of wood but with a metal grill. A small heap of moxa is placed on the grill and lit so that it glows red hot. The box is then placed on the patient's body (frequently on the stomach or back). An intensive warmth spreads and a thin film of oil from the moxa forms on the skin. A moxa box can't be used in the ear.

Moxa sticks are made up of hard-packed moxa, rolled in thin paper, like a thick cigarette. There are sticks made of pure moxa, others in which it is blended with other healing herbs and so-called smokeless moxa, hard sticks that emit less smoke than the usual ones.

In body acupuncture, a piece of a moxa stick is fastened to an acupuncture needle (see Fig. 9.11). When it is lighted it warms both the needle and the skin. A lighted moxa stick may also be held over the skin to warm it. In ear acupuncture

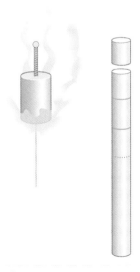

Figure 9.11 Moxa.

it is too risky to fasten moxa to the needle because of the danger of glowing embers so close to the hair. If an ordinary moxa stick is used, it is difficult to warm a specific point because the stick is too thick. So-called 'tiger warmers', thinner moxa sticks, more like incense sticks, made of moxa, cinnamon and other herbs, are easier to use in the ears.

Triangular needles and lancets

Triangular needles were formerly most often used to induce bleeding. These are thick needles with a three-edged tip. The idea was that a few drops of blood would seep out. Nowadays it is more common to use a lancet of the type used in taking blood samples from fingertips.

Laser

Nogier differentiated between auriculotherapy (regular ear acupuncture) and auriculomedicine, which is a more advanced form of ear treatment. Auriculomedicine makes use of more technically advanced apparatus, including lasers. Nogier worked out a programme for laser treatment of the ear's zones. He created three programmes for treatment of the ear. These are preprogrammed into the lasers used in auriculomedicine. They are named Regeneration, Muscle Relaxation and Antalgic (pain relieving).

10

Examination of the ear

Chapter contents

Before you start using ear acupuncture

Ear acupuncture is a simple and safe method which, on its own or in combination with other forms of healthcare is effective in treating many different painful conditions and ailments. However, there are other illnesses for which ear acupuncture is an unsuitable form of treatment. A basic medical education makes it easier to judge which conditions should not be treated. Certain symptoms must be treated by a doctor.

I work on the assumption that the patient has been examined by a doctor who has ruled out serious illness or one that requires another form of treatment. To camouflage symptoms that need another form of treatment can be fatal. For example, the ear acupuncturist should not take away pain that might be an alarm for a condition requiring an operation. Use your common sense. Be serious, promise no more than the method can deliver and don't pretend that you know more than you do. Refer a patient needing other treatment to someone who can provide them with that treatment.

You should, for a start, have taken a course in ear acupuncture. It's a plus to have access to a supervisor. It can be an advantage to be able to put questions to someone well versed in ear acupuncture if you are at all unsure. Practise on volunteer adults in your immediate circle until you feel sure you have mastered the technique.

As with other forms of treatment: be sure to keep the times you have booked for your patients. Waiting creates irritation in patients and it will be more difficult for you to judge their condition as a result. Make sure too that you yourself are calm, relaxed and have slept well so you can give of your best.

Equipment

The equipment absolutely necessary for ear acupuncture will fit into a pocket — needles, alcohol swabs and cotton buds. If you invest in a mechanical point detector too you will have a better chance of finding the right points. With an electrical point detector there will be an even better possibility of providing optimum treatment.

Prepare yourself before meeting the patient. Read up on the method, think about the symptoms displayed by the patient so you know where to begin looking for active points.

You'll need a good textbook on ear acupuncture and a detailed poster showing the points in the ear. It's a good idea to have such a poster on the wall so you can demonstrate the reflex system and the treatment you propose for your patients, if they are interested. If you find it necessary to look up many things in your textbook during treatment, you'll communicate your uncertainty to the patient, who may with good reason start wondering if you know what you are doing.

A practice rubber or silicon ear can be good to have if you want to show the patient what you are about to do. Plus you can use it in the pauses between patients to practise the agility of your fingers until you have a really superb needle technique.

You should think about what you should do with the used needles. They are counted as dangerous waste and should not be dumped with your ordinary household garbage. If you work in the health service or for some other body that has a functioning system for the collection of dangerous waste, place your acupuncture needles in the same container as that for sampling and injection needles. If you work in a clinic without a system for needle disposal containers, contact your local authority and ask for advice on disposal.

Be prepared

Begin the examination by making sure you have everything you'll need within easy reach. It's unprofessional to leave the patient midway through the examination and start looking for something you need.

Check that your fingernails are short and clean. Wash your hands.

Lay out the things you'll need for ear acupuncture on a tray or a table

You'll need:

- alcohol swabs
- a mechanical probe
- an electrical point detector (if you have access to one)
- regular acupuncture needles (about 0.20 × 13 mm)
- cotton buds to wipe away drops of blood
- semi-permanent needles
- pellets and seeds (on band aid)
- tweezers to use when putting in press tacks and to remove semi-permanent needles
- a container for dangerous waste for used needles.

Within reach you will also need:

- disposal bin for blood-stained rubbish (dangerous waste)
- waste paper basket for other rubbish.

Other things that can be good to have around when you start treatment:

- your glasses
- a journal
- a pen that works
- a torch or a strap-on forehead lamp if you have poor lighting.

The room

The premises where you receive your patients should be appropriate for what you are going to do, clean and pleasant so that the patients relax and have trust in you. There should be a washbasin in the vicinity so that you can quickly and frequently wash your hands. The room should be easy to keep clean, well ventilated and have good lighting. A toilet for patients is a must.

You don't need to purchase advanced examination benches or chairs. The patient can lie on a simple bench or bed which is a suitable height for you. The patient can also sit up during the examination and treatment. In NADA treatment (a standardised form of ear acupuncture given to treat addiction, see Ch. 13, NADA – using ear acupuncture to fight addiction) it is customary for the patients to sit in a group. Ordinary chairs are acceptable, though those with arm rests are best. If the chair is not sufficiently high backed so that the patient can lean back and rest the neck during treatment you can stand it next to a wall with a cushion or pillow between. If you want things a little more *de luxe*, add an armchair with a footrest or a chair with an adjustable back. Baden-Baden-type garden furniture is usually quite suitable.

If patients are scared it is best for them to lie down during the first sessions to lessen the risk of them fainting. (Fainting is a very unusual side effect in ear acupuncture. See Ch. 11, Method.)

Starting the examination

Shake your new patient by the hand, look them in the eye and welcome them.[1]

You can gain a great deal of information about patients, even when they are in the waiting room. Are they worried, restless, abnormally tired or stressed?

Take a few minutes to try to 'read' your patients, to show them they are welcome and try to get on their wavelengths so that you can cooperate with them.

Keeping a journal

Take careful case histories of your patients, write a journal. Authorised healthcare personnel have to write journals and others can benefit from the practice, even if they don't *have* to. Write down what you do and why you do it. The next time you

---

[1] It has been shown that patients being treated with antibiotics for tonsillitis have a better rate of healing if the doctor shakes hands with them than if there is no such physical contact. Take advantage of all such simple measures to boost the chance of obtaining a positive result of treatment.

have contact with the patient note what has happened since the first treatment. Much later it can be worthwhile to be able to refer to the journal and see what it was you did that time when the symptoms disappeared — or what you did when there was no satisfactory result.

Take a history:

- On the first encounter start by briefly asking patients their reasons for seeking treatment.
- Note name, date of birth, address, telephone number, marital status and ask about occupation. (Conditions at work or in the home may be contributory factors to the illness.) Is the patient on sick-leave? Does the patient have a medical certificate to be off work? If so, is it temporary or long term? What was the diagnosis given by the doctor on the certificate?
- Ask more about the patient's symptoms. How did the illness start? How has it developed? If the patient is experiencing pain, make a sketch of the body and fill in the affected areas. Ask what brings on the pain, and what makes it better.
- What examinations, treatment, operations or hospital visits have there been? This can help you make a prognosis. Someone who has already tried every sort of treatment imaginable, who has been operated on and perhaps ingested medicine over a long period has less chance of successful treatment than someone who has recently fallen ill. It can still be worth trying ear acupuncture but you will not need to feel as if you have failed because you too have been unable to solve the problem.
- Find out about the patient's medication. Consider whether the patient's symptoms could be related to that medication.
- Ask about other illnesses the patient has or has had.
- Try to build a picture of the patient's general energy level, in relation to age and illness. One way to do this can be to ask, 'Do you feel more tired than you think you should be considering your circumstances?'
- Take blood pressure and pulse rate if relevant.
- Try to walk a middle line in allowing chatty patients to talk freely about their condition, while at the same time keeping charge of the questioning so that you obtain a clear picture of how the patient feels.

You need to note which points in the ear are active, which points you treat and how you treat each one of them (if you use a regular acupuncture needle, a semi-permanent needle, a pellet or whether you treated the patient in some other way).

After a telephone inquiry you should write down what the patient says concerning symptoms or why he or she has cancelled their appointment.

Right- or left-handed?

On the first visit you should take note of whether the patient is right-handed, left-handed or is concealing his or her left-handedness. The latter is someone who is really left-handed but who uses the right hand because they have learned to do so.

According to the Nogier school of thought, such people can have laterality problems and should be treated for these before treatment is administered for anything else. See Laterality in Ch. 5.

To discover a patient's laterality, Nogier recommends these tests

- Ask your patient to pretend to take a photo. The eye used to look into the camera with will be on the dominant side.
- Push your standing patient backwards. His dominant leg will first be moved backwards to protect him from falling.
- Note which hand the patient uses to gesticulate with in emphasising what it is he or she is saying. This provides a clear indication of the dominant side.
- Note which shoulder is held highest, another indication of the dominant side.
- Shake both your patient's hands. The grip will be strongest on the dominant side.

By finding out whether the patient is right- or left-handed, you'll also discover which ear is dominant, something that determines something in which ear you'll have best effect if you don't want to use the functional points in both ears. On right-handed people it is the right ear that is dominant and vice versa.

Other questions

If you are interested in Nogier's method of treatment you should also ask about other things, such as scars, diet and condition of the teeth. (See Therapy blockage in Ch. 11 page 167).

Is other treatment necessary?

Consider whether the patient may need other treatment or examination (such as surgery, medicine, chiropractic manipulation, x-ray examination, blood test, psychotherapy or counselling). If so refer the patient to the relevant practitioner.

If you consider that ear acupuncture is a suitable treatment for your patient you can outline your prognosis, how much treatment you think will be required and how often you should see the patient. If you decide that treatment is appropriate you can begin to examine the ear and look for active points.

Suggestions for your journal

In your journal, in addition to mapping out a case history (see Fig. 10.1), you should also note which points are active during your examination, which points you chose to treat and how you treated them (see Fig. 10.2).

Looking for active points

Begin by washing your hands. Explain to your patient that you are about to look for active points and that you would like to know about any points that they feel to be sore.

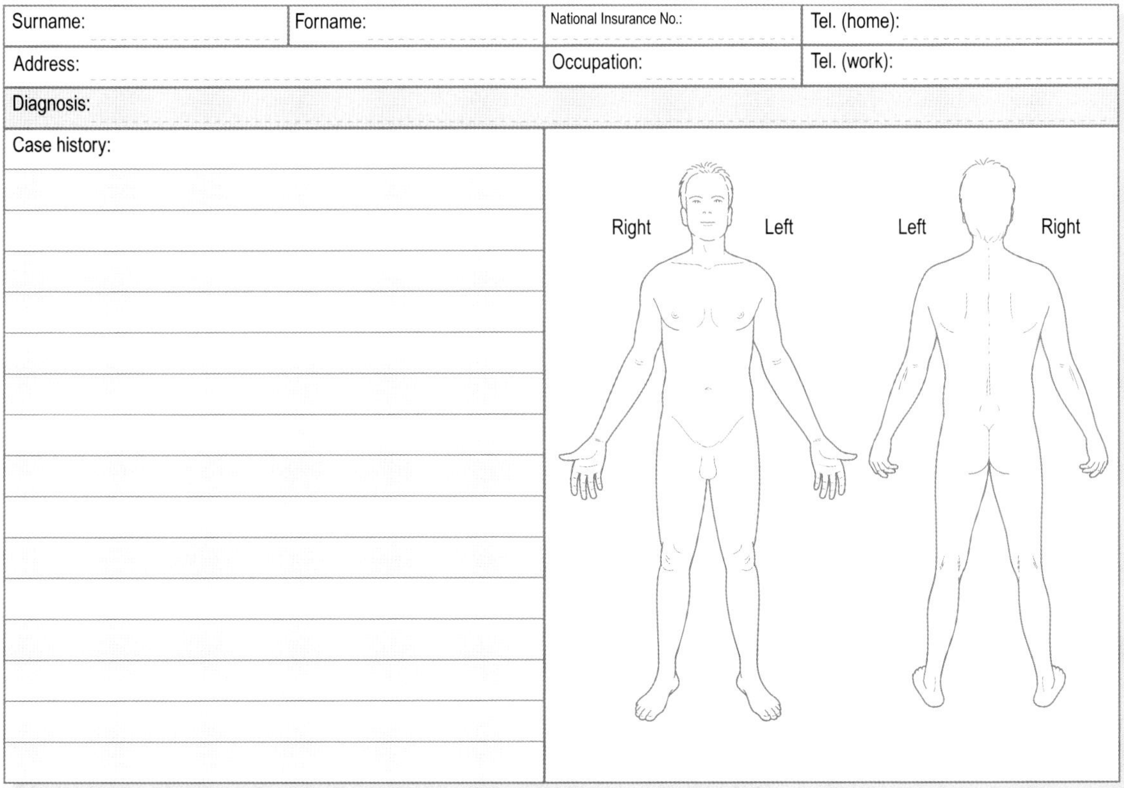

Surname:	Forname:	National Insurance No.:	Tel. (home):
Address:		Occupation:	Tel. (work):
Diagnosis:			

Case history:

Right   Left   Left   Right

Figure 10.1 On a page in your journal make use of sketches on which you can pencil in the patient's symptoms, for example the spread of pain.

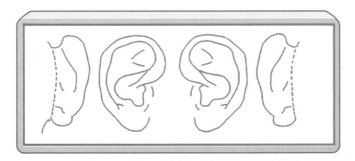

Figure 10.2 It is useful to have a picture of the ear in your journal on which to mark active and treated points. A rubber stamp of an ear, such as the one in the picture, can make this job easier.

Take your time when examining the patient's ear. Care in examination is vital in determining treatment. Start where points matching the patient's symptoms should be according to the reflex map, then look for active points among the functional points. Don't forget to also search for active points more distal to Point Zero, for example in the scaphoid fossa, in the vegetative groove and at the helix (see Ch. 12, page 171 for Point Zero geometry, the radius system).

Position yourself so you can work in a relaxed fashion. You'll do a better job if your shoulders and arms are relaxed, both when you examine the ear and when you treat it.

Avoid twisting or holding on to the patient's head to get it in the right position during your examination. It can be unpleasant, even insulting, to be 'corrected' by having your head twisted to the right position. It's better to ask patients to turn their heads themselves. In this way you generate a feeling that the two of you are cooperating to achieve optimum working conditions.

Good lighting can also be decisive in achieving good results. Make sure you have a fair amount of daylight coming from windows, a light that you can turn so that it is focused on the ear, a torch or a strap-on forehead lamp.

The patient can lie on a couch with a little cushion as support for the head. (Large, soft cushions have a tendency to fluff up and conceal the ears, which would make examination more difficult and increase the likelihood of needles more easily coming loose during treatment.) Sit behind your patient's headrest with the tray or table containing your equipment within easy reach so that you can work peacefully and calmly with your patient's ears.

An alternative is that the patient should sit up during the examination. You can either sit on a chair alongside or stand, if that gives you a better working position. If you decide to work standing up, it can be good to have your patient sitting on an office chair which can be raised or lowered. (The patient can move to a more comfortable chair when the needles are in place.)

Inspection

First look carefully at the ear. Examine its appearance before you clean the ear, touch or 'disturb' it in some other way. Practise noticing changes in colour.

Are there marks, knots, unusual structures or visible blood vessels? Make a note of where they are. Such signs can mean that there are disturbances in the organs that are reflected in the corresponding part of the ear.

Search too for colour changes or changed pigmentation. An area that is paler, redder or darker and which changes colour under palpation is a positive sign, indicating that there is an active point.

Colour changes

According to traditional Chinese medicine (TCM, see Ch. 2, A brief look at traditional Chinese medicine), pale zones mean that the corresponding organ is suffering a deficiency in qi or blood (deficiency in Chinese is known as xu-condition), impaired circulation. It can be an old wound or a chronic organic disease. For example, arthritis can give rise to a paleness in the zone that corresponds to the afflicted part of the body.

Redder zones may mean that the corresponding organ has an excess (excess in Chinese is known as shi-condition). In other words it is over-functioning. The excess condition may express itself in the form of an infection, heat, stagnation or a strong pain. For example, tonsillitis can give rise to red dots on the tonsil points on the helix. The red zones become manifest often in the case of conditions that are either acute or subacute and are important points for treatment.

A visible blood vessel may often appear in a zone in the ear corresponding to a damaged organ. Changes to the skin of the ear in the form of white flakes or secretion which cannot easily be wiped away are worth observing. A heightened activity in the specific sympathetic nerves controlling the flow of blood can lead to a microscopic contraction of blood vessels in corresponding zones, causing cell damage on a small area of the ear.

Freckles or blackheads don't indicate an active point and shouldn't influence your diagnosis.

The form of the ear

According to TCM, it is possible to judge a person's constitution by the position and form of the ear. The upper edge of the ear is usually on a level with the corner of the eye. Ears that are very low can be a sign of mental deficiencies. According to TCM, a well-formed ear with a clearly marked lobe indicates wisdom and a good constitution. Buddha is often portrayed with elongated earlobes as a sign of his great wisdom. People with large earlobes are said to be wise and plan for their future. They cultivate faith instead of fear. People with large earlobes have the ability to grow things — people, plants, animals or investments, writes Bridges in her book *Face Reading* (2004). She claims that people with small earlobes tend to live in the present and do not focus on their future.

According to TCM the size of the ears are related to courage and risk-taking ability. Bridges writes: 'Large ears often belong to gamblers' and 'Small ears belong to cautious and careful people'. If the ear is broad across the top the person is more capable of taking mental or financial risks, and if the ear is broad across the middle it indicates that the person is capable of taking physical risks.

50-year crease

People who have reached 50 often have a little crease in the skin in front of the tragus (see Fig. 10.3). In forensic medicine, for example, the crease is used to determine a person's age.

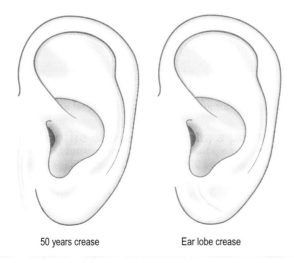

50 years crease   Ear lobe crease

Figure 10.3 50-year crease Earlobe crease.

The earlobe crease

A crease of the lobe of the ear, running from the incisura intertragica straight downwards or sloping diagonally backwards over the lobe, indicates a greater risk for heart or vascular illness (Fig. 10.3). If the crease is there from birth it means nothing, but if it comes about later in life (most often at an age of around 35), comprehensive studies have shown a close connection between this crease and heart and cardiovascular disease. People who have the crease should be motivated to lessen the risk of illness by eliminating other risk factors such as smoking, stress, obesity and poor diet.

Deformed ears

If children in the West are born with deformed ears, an examination of the kidneys is often made because a clear statistical connection has been shown to exist between deformed ears and defective kidneys. (According to TCM, the kidneys 'open' in the ear and ancient texts refer to a connection between the ear and the kidney.)

Wounds that can be seen in the ear

If a part of the body is subjected to a trauma, for example an athletic injury, a red blood vessel may become visible in the part of the ear corresponding to the damaged body part soon after the accident.

In cases of chronic damage the part of the ear corresponding to the injured organ can be seen to change form.

Feel with your fingers

When you have looked at the ears, it is time to touch them. Take your time. This exercise can provide you with a great deal of information. Besides which, it is a way of getting close to the patient and gently starting the treatment.

According to TCM you can get information about the inherited constitution by touching the ear. Bridges (2004) writes: 'Evaluate the strength of the cartilage. Firm ears indicate strength in the kidneys and a healthy constitution. They are indicative of good *jing*. They should not be too stiff, however. The best ears are flexible but have some tensile strength, like *al dente* pasta. Ears that are too stiff indicate a propensity to high blood pressure and ears that are too flimsy, thin and transparent belong to people with weak constitutions'.

Palpate with thumb and forefinger. Does it feel 'grainy', as if there was grain of sand under the skin? Can you, even at this stage, provoke a grimace? 'The grimace sign' (when the patient gives a start, blinks or in some other way shows an involuntary reaction) is far more reliable than asking whether it hurts.

Note the location of the change/soreness.

Massage

It can be a good idea not just to feel with the fingers but to give a massage. If the patient has come in from the cold just before the treatment the ears can be warmed by massaging them. It can happen that the acupuncturist encourages the patient to massage the ears before the needles are inserted. The aim of this is put the focus on the ears and to calm and prepare patients for treatment.

A disadvantage with massage before acupuncture is that one can 'massage away' positive signs. Positive signs seen before the massage, for example reddening, pallor or secretion in a particular zone, can disappear.

Massage of the ears can also be a form of treatment. A more systematic massage of the ear is described on page 159.

Looking for active points with your probe

Now it is time to feel all the different zones of the ear in a more careful manner. The fundamental principle of ear acupuncture is to find and treat active points. Finding active points can be decisive when it comes to achieving results. Look carefully, let your examination take the time needed.

You need an object to palpate — feel around — the ear with. You can use a mechanical probe or a more advanced electric point detector (see pages 125–127).

On the rest of the body all the acupuncture points are constantly active. You can locate them at any time with a point detector. In the ear the only active points, in addition to the master points, are those corresponding to a damaged body part or an impaired function. This is one of the fundamental differences between the two forms of acupuncture.

Take your time and be systematic

Take your time and be systematic as you examine both ears. Ask about soreness or trust to the 'grimace sign' — those times a patient gives an involuntary grimace when you touch an active point. Perhaps the patient will blink or the corner of the mouth will twitch. Assure yourself that the patient has understood that you are looking for active points and needs to inform you where there is sensitivity. But remember 'the grimace sign' is likely to be a much more reliable indicator than the patient describing the sensation in a point verbally.

Search for active points by pushing the probe over the skin. Be careful to use the same pressure and to search equally long in each zone. If you use a spring-loaded probe, be careful not to press too hard. Let the pen glide over the surface of the ear. Support the rear of the patient's ear with one finger of your free hand when, for example, you're looking in the scaphoid fossa or the edge of the helix. Be careful when you are searching close to the outer ear canal. A slip there can be very unpleasant for the patient. To avoid this you can cover the ear canal with a fingertip while you search for active points in the area.

A probe which at one end resembles a screwdriver or a stirrup is excellent for searching the raised parts of the ear, for example the helix root or the edge along the antihelix. If you search for the sore point corresponding to a painful vertebra and drag the 'screwdriver' or 'stirrup' along the zone where the vertebra is represented, it's easy to find the exact point. If the flat part of the tool is dragged gently along the helix root, it will sink easily down into the crease containing Point Zero.

If you don't have a probe, you can use a simpler tool. Try turning a regular acupuncture needle and palpating with the end of the handle (only be careful not to contaminate the tip of the needle), or try the end of a match, the flat end of a toothpick, an old ballpoint pen, a small crochet hook or some other blunt object. The flat end of a paperclip can substitute for a 'screwdriver' pressure pen.

Both under-active and over-active points can be sore (when it comes to under-active points, it may take a little longer before the patient experiences pain). Note where it is sore and where the pressure pen sinks down or creates an indentation. (When it is time for treatment, a needle can be inserted in the indentation.)

Use just the right pressure

Don't be too eager and cause pain. If you push hard and long enough on the same point it will become painful even if it isn't active. Search as objectively and with as open a mind as possible.

Be sure that your shoulders and arms are relaxed while you carry out the examination and take good time about it. You're looking for the points you will be treating. It's important to get it right.

Clean the probe with alcohol after use.

Electrical point detectors

If you have access to an electrical point detector (see Ch. 9, Equipment) you'll get exact information as to where the active points in the ear are located.

Wipe the ear with alcohol in good time for the examination, so the alcohol has had time to evaporate. This takes some minutes. If the ear is damp the instrument will show too many active points. It can be a good idea to clean the patient's ear even before you conduct your interview.

If the ear has been treated with skin lotion (for example foundation make up), this must be cleaned away before the examination, partly so the instrument will measure correctly, partly to protect the tip of the point detector from unnecessary fat.

There are different types of point detector. Read the instructions and try out your point detector on someone you know so you're sure of how it will work when you use it on your patients. If you show uncertainty in handling the instrument and its connections, the patient may lose confidence in your abilities.

Begin by calibrating the instrument according to the instruction booklet. Usually this will be based on the resistance at Point Zero, but some instruments may be calibrated from the ear lobe. Then begin your search. It is important to use equal pressure and time for all points. The probe should be held at a right angle to the ear and only the tip should move against the skin. Search slowly and systematically in both ears by drawing the point detector across the skin.

When an electrical point detector comes into contact with an active point a lamp will blink or there will be a warning beep. This is how you know you've found an active point. If your instrument can transmit you can also treat the point by pushing a button and send a weak stream of current into the active point.

Do not put blind faith in instruments. If you don't get the answer you expected from the point detector, it's sensible to look for technical faults. Make sure the batteries are working, that the probe is clean and (if you are using an instrument connected with wires) that there are no loose contacts. The most common fault when using simpler types of point detector which do not require the patient to hold a probe is that the acupuncturist's free hand loses contact with the patient (in which case the instrument stops working) or that a protruding part of the ear has moved against some part of the probe (causing the pen to give a false reading).

When the point detector locates a point it very often will leave a mark making it easy to see exactly where to insert the needle.

Clean the point detector with alcohol after use.

Which ear should you examine for active points?

If the patient has a complaint on one particular side of the body, there is an 80 percent chance of finding active points in the ear on the same side. In 20 percent of cases the corresponding active point will be in the ear on the opposite side or in both ears. If you look for an active point for the elbow of a patient with an injury to the left elbow, it's most likely that you will find the point in the left ear. If you don't, look in the equivalent zone in the right ear.

Certain organs are, like functional points, not right- or left-sided. The large intestine lies to both left and right of the body. Active points for it can be found in the right and/or left ear.

Allergies and hormonal disturbances are not situated on one or another side of the body. First search for the functional point in the dominant ear. The right ear is reckoned to be dominant on a right-handed person and the left on a left-handed person.

How the degree of soreness relates to the seriousness of the complaint

The soreness of the point in the ear is not in proportion to the degree of seriousness of the illness. It is important to inform worried patients of this. If many points are sore and perhaps are really painful under palpation, the patient can interpret the pain by thinking there is something seriously wrong and feel worse as a result. If a point is sore, the acupuncturist merely draws the conclusion that it is active and that there is a disturbance in the corresponding part of the body or of a function but does not reach any conclusion as to how serious it might be.

Active points may change place

An active point can change place from day to day, sometimes even during consultation. It can even change ears. Because the points are to a certain degree mobile, you must be flexible, observant and without preconceived ideas. Therefore you should not conduct treatment only by following a point map but treat each ear individually and choose the points in it that are active. There is no ready-made formula for ear acupuncture.

Note in your journal which points were active during the examination, which points you chose to treat and how you treated them.

Marking the points and applying acupressure

Palpation of the ear takes place as part of an examination but this can also be a form of treatment. If you find an active point and let the point detector stay on the point, you can perform acupressure (using pressure on the point rather than inserting a needle). It can be rewarding to make use of this effect when you have been successful in finding an active point: just let the point detector linger on the point for a few seconds (see page 159).

If after the examination you intend to treat with acupuncture (the most usual treatment), the point detector will now have made a small indentation in the active point, making it easy to see exactly where the needle should be inserted.

However, it is not a good idea to mark active points with a colour pen. If you do so and then prick your patients you risk tattooing them, because the colour particles may follow the needle down into the skin.

What if you find no active points?

When the patient describes his or her symptoms during your introductory interview you can take a guess at where the active points are likely to be found. With any luck, you'll find them quickly. Sometimes the opposite may be true: the ear is 'dumb' and there are no active points to be found. In such a case start searching in the same zones in the other ear. Twenty percent of patients have active points in the ear on the opposite side to the ailment. If you find no active points, ask the patient to massage the ears and then try again.

Some authors recommend the acupuncturist to insert a needle, preferably a gold one, in Point Zero if the ear is 'dumb'. After around a quarter of an hour, you can begin searching again for active points.

As a last resort, if you find no active points, treat the zones of the ear according to a point map, inserting needles where the points should be. But the best results are obtained by finding the active points. (Read more on the choice of points in Ch. 12, Treatment Suggestions.)

Method

When the acupuncturist has examined the ear and found one or more active points, it is time to decide which points should be treated and how. A point can be worked on in many different ways: with acupuncture needles, pellets and seeds, massage, acupressure, electricity, by being bled or by being radiated with light or a laser beam. In practice regular acupuncture needles, semi-permanent needles and pellets of different types are most commonly used.

In this chapter we will look at different methods of ear acupuncture treatment. We will also look at exactly what can be treated, contraindications, side effects and therapy hindrances. How to choose the points to be treated, and suggestions for treatment based on different indications, will be described in Ch. 12, Treatment suggestions.

Lessening the risk of infection

Alcohol swabs have been used to clean the skin before injections or acupuncture to lessen the risk of infection. But wiping the skin with an alcohol swab does not mean that the area thus treated becomes sterile. The alcohol dries quickly and does not have time to kill all micro-organisms. Besides, many micro-organisms are found not on the skin but inside and under it. These 'hidden' microbes are not affected when the surface is cleaned with a swab.

Nowadays many injections are given without first wiping the skin with alcohol. Acupuncture needles are of a much smaller diameter than syringes, which makes them less likely to carry bacteria into the tissue.

A British medical journal published in 2001 an article with a precise overview of criteria concerning cleansing the skin before acupuncture (Hoffman 2001). The author's conclusion was that wiping with alcohol of a normally clean skin before an injection or acupuncture was partially ineffective (the bacteria stay put) and moreover unnecessary. The likelihood of a thin, sterile acupuncture needle causing infection in a patient without an immune deficiency disorder is, according to the author, very remote. However, if the skin is visibly dirty, it should be washed with soap and water before acupuncture treatment.

Hand washing

I must emphasise the importance of acupuncturists practising good hand hygiene. In the article referred to above it is pointed out that acupuncturists should wash their hands with soap and water, or rinse them in an alcohol solution before starting treatment. Even microscopically small amounts of tissue fluid can spread disease from one person to another. The hepatitis B virus can move from one patient to another in 10 pL serum (1 pL = 0.000000001 mL).

Disposable needles lessen risk of infection

In the fight against infection, the use of disposable needles is more important than cleaning with alcohol swabs. The greatest risk of infection in acupuncture occurred in years gone by when needles were used several times and sterilised between sessions. If the sterilisation was not handled properly the hepatitus virus, to give one example, could survive and spread among patients.

Why care must be taken in the ear

While cleaning with alcohol swabs may not be favoured in body acupuncture, in ear acupuncture one can never be too careful in my opinion. In the ear needles are inserted in or near cartilage, which has poorer blood circulation than other tissue and thus poorer healing capacity. An infection in cartilage is difficult to cure and may require treatment with intravenous antibiotics.

Taking care when using semi-permanent needles

The risk of infection is greater if you use semi-permanent needles. They stay put in the ear for several days, creating a way through the skin to underlying tissue.

Despite the fact that semi-permanent needles are used so frequently, accidents are rare. Arne J Norheim (1994), a Norwegian doctor, in an article in a medical journal listed acupuncture complications from all over the world. During the period 1981–1992 there were 10 reported cases of cartilage infection after ear acupuncture described on the Medline database. 'Intravenous antibiotic treatment and in some cases drainage meant that only two of the patients developed necrosis and deformities' wrote Norheim.

Bearing in mind how many millions of acupuncture needles were in use in the world during the period in question this is a remarkably low accident rate. Nevertheless, one should be extra observant when using semi-permanent needles and I recommend wiping with alcohol swabs in such cases.

If semi-permanent needles are used, it is also important to inform patients about the risk of infection and what they should do if they suspect they have caught one (see page 157).

Isopropyl alcohol

Ready-made, disposable injection swabs soaked in 70 percent isopropyl alcohol may be used. They are easy to use but a little more expensive than making your own. Ready-made swabs also create more garbage.

An alternative is to use non-sterile compresses dampened in alcohol solution. They are cheaper and reduce unnecessary packaging.

Other good reasons for wiping with alcohol

Even if it is unnecessary for bacteriological reasons to wipe the ear with alcohol before acupuncture treatment, there can be other good grounds for getting into the habit of routinely cleaning the ear in this way:

- you communicate a feeling of care, responsibility and professionalism and show that your clinic has a good standard of hygiene
- it's a good way of starting the treatment and an easy way of getting close to the patient
- while you're wiping the ear you will have time to note its structure and colouring
- the contact will make many patients feel good
- on some patients visible dirt will have to be cleaned from the ear. The patient can be in such bad shape that he or she cannot be bothered with personal hygiene. Patients sometimes take part in daily ear acupuncture sessions, in a group (for example, NADA is a standardised form of ear acupuncture given daily to patients with addiction problems, see Ch. 13). If everyone's ears are wiped, you will not have the embarrassing task of picking out individuals who are so dirty that cleaning is a necessity.
- blood stains can be left over from a previous treatment. Bacteria thrives in blood so it is important to wash away old blood before inserting a new needle
- if you wipe the patient's ears, your hands will be kept clean at the same time by the alcohol
- if you choose to let patients wipe their own ears with an alcohol swab, you will give them the feeling that they are taking part in the treatment and capable of taking responsibility for themselves
- if you use a point detector, wiping the ear with alcohol swabs helps to prevent the probe from getting dirty with grease and sediment.

Stimulating the point

While you examined the ear, chose which points to treat, marked them so that a small indentation was formed and wiped the ear with alcohol, you should have had time to ponder over a suitable method of treatment. You'll have chosen between inserting regular acupuncture needles, semi-permanent needles, pellets, treatment with electricity or laser, or administering acupressure by pressing on the points.

If both ear acupuncture and body acupuncture are being administered in the same treatment, you can start with either one or the other.

Needle technique for regular ear acupuncture

In ear acupuncture the idea is that the needles just penetrate the skin to a depth of around 2 mm. This is why not much force is needed for the initial penetration. The ear acupuncturist strives for a very limited and soft movement of the fingers to insert the needle in as pain free a fashion as possible.[1]

---

[1] A person who is more familiar with body acupuncture uses greater force when inserting needles than that which is necessary in ear acupuncture. Often the body acupuncturist makes an initial chopping movement with the wrist to get the needle into the skin quickly. Afterwards a gentler movement is used to drive the needle the rest of the way until the desired depth is reached.

Hold the needle with two or three fingers. The tip of the needle which is to be inserted in the skin must of course be kept sterile. The fingers should be held in a softly rounded position, holding the needle at an angle of around 45 degrees against the index finger. If the needle is held parallel with the index finger your fine motor skills will be impaired and it will be difficult for you to perform the small movements necessary for smooth, pain-free insertion.

Small, gentle movement

No great force is needed to get the needle to the right depth (1–3 mm). Use just the fingers, not your wrist and absolutely not your elbow or shoulder to push in the needle. Insert with a gentle movement. If the ear acupuncturist uses the wrist in a chopping motion, this will cause real pain, even if the needle is driven only a few millimetres into the skin.

Insert firmly, but gently. Lay the tip of the needle very close to the skin and then drive it in with a decided but gentle movement. (If you first lay the needle so that the tip touches the skin and then push it in, pain reflexes will be triggered twice, which is unnecessary.)

Practise your insertion technique using an object before you try with people, for example a practice ear made of rubber and silicon. Such practice ears are useful for learning to find your way around the ear and for demonstrating to the patient how the treatment is to be carried out.

Support the hand you use for inserting the needle against the patient. Support your little finger up against the patient's head or cheek. Avoid touching and moving the patient's head in any other way — this may be experienced as unpleasant and insulting.

To rotate or not to rotate?

Often the needle is driven through the skin with a rotating movement. According to traditional Chinese medicine (TCM), the direction in which the needle is rotated when it is inserted and the intensity with which it is manipulated have an effect on the efficacy of the treatment. One can tonify by rotating the needle clockwise and using small movements. Should you want to spread the energy instead, the needle should be rotated anticlockwise and manipulated with more powerful movements. The same idea is sometimes used in ear acupuncture[2] but it matters less in which direction the needle is rotated, more that it has been placed in the right point and will stay inserted long enough to have an effect. Because the needle is inserted about 2 mm it is also technically difficult to manipulate it, so many ear acupuncturists choose instead to insert needles in 'neutral' fashion, straight in, with a gentle movement.

According to certain schools it is important in which order the needles are inserted and taken out. However, most acupuncturists believe this really doesn't matter a great deal.

---

[2] For example, in NADA acupuncture (ear acupuncture used to treat addiction, see Ch. 13) the needle is rotated clockwise during insertion. There are several reasons for this. Partly the initial puncture is less painful if the needle is rotated. (In NADA acupuncture it is more important that treatment should be pain-free because some of the patients who receive the treatment will have a lower pain threshold as a result of drug abuse.) In addition in traditional Chinese medicine the belief is that drugs drain the user of qi (energy) and of yin (See Ch. 2, A brief look at traditional Chinese medicine (TCM)). By rotating the needle clockwise it is thought that one tonifies, adds, that which is missing.

Which direction?

As a rule acupuncture needles are inserted at right angles to the skin's surface. In this way you'll find only one point with each needle. If the needle is inserted obliquely into the skin you risk threading several points with the same needle. An exception to right angle insertion is when you 'tunnel', pull the needle as if it were in a tunnel under the skin, to deliberately hit more than one point.

For example: In childbirth when seeking to give the greatest pain relief possible for a limited duration, the acupuncturist can 'tunnel' by inserting a needle linking the points Shen Men and Uterus. Or if a patient has pain in an arm, for example after a stroke, you can tunnel a needle in the scaphoid fossa so that a greater part of the zone that corresponds to the arm is stimulated.

How deep?

The needle need not go deeper than 1–3 mm. The needle should stand steady and straight and not fall out when the patient moves his head. Many ear acupuncturists at the start of their careers are afraid to cause the patient any discomfort and can be overly careful when inserting needles. In such cases it often happens that the needles fall out before the treatment period is up. If the handle of the needle hangs down or dangles, then you know that you should apply more pressure next time you make an insertion.

On the other hand, the ear is very thin in certain places. It is relatively easy to stick a needle right through, so that the tip comes out on the other side of the ear. This should not happen. The tip of the needle, which at that point is no longer sterile, may transport bacteria with it when it is removed. If it does happen, carefully draw the needle back to the right depth and for safety's sake clean the area with alcohol afterwards.

Pinch…

Inform the patient that the insertion may hurt so he or she won't be surprised. Say that you are going to pinch the ear to divert the pain. Pinch the ear with your free hand and insert the needle with the other.

Use both hands in this way in ear acupuncture until you are so experienced that you're 100 percent sure of being able to make the insertion without causing pain. Take a proper grip of the ear, so hard that the pinch diverts the pain the patient would otherwise feel from the insertion. Pinch without pulling at the ear. To pull someone's ear can be experienced as an unpleasant means of correction and it also temporarily displaces the ear's topography.

take a deep breath…

Pain is experienced differently during inhalation and exhalation. It is most intense when you hold your breath. If the needle is inserted during exhalation it will cause demonstrably less discomfort. Therefore always try to seize the opportunity to insert the needle when the patient is exhaling.[3] Demonstrate the correlation of

---

[3] According to certain ancient texts in TCM, the body acupuncturist should insert the needle when the patient is inhaling if the aim is to tonify and when the patient is exhaling if the aim is to sedate. Other such texts state the reverse. In ear acupuncture, in which the insertion is more superficial and faster than in body acupuncture, the direction of rotation during insertion is most likely of less importance.

breathing and the insertion of the needles before you begin if the patient is in the least bit nervous or afraid that the treatment will be painful. Show the patient first how to breathe in then how to exhale, the latter more forcefully and faster. Then ask the patient to take a deep breath as you concentrate on getting the tip of the needle so close to the point that the tip is practically touching the skin.

...and insert!

Then, while the patient breathes out, insert the needle, gently and calmly. Don't force it. Lay the tip of the needle close to the point and push it in with the gentle, decided motion we talked about earlier.

How does it feel?

When the needle pierces the skin, the patient will of course feel it. However, it is unusual for patients to experience the pain as being so off-putting that they decide against any further ear acupuncture sessions. The pain of insertion can to a large degree be diminished with good needle technique, by pinching the patient's ear and by making the insertion when the patient is exhaling.

In ear acupuncture 'de qi' (see Ch. 2, A brief look at traditional Chinese medicine) is not a sought after effect, as it is in body acupuncture. The needles are therefore usually not stimulated during treatment. You insert the needle and leave it there. Nevertheless, sometimes the patient will experience a form of 'de qi'. The ear may feel warm, it may feel as if the ear has grown larger, or the ear may redden.

Stimulating the needles

In cases where a painful condition is being treated, stimulation of the needles increases the possibility of achieving rapid relief. In such cases the needles are manipulated (either rotated or vibrated) at regular intervals during treatment. Another option is electrical stimulation of the needles (see further on in this chapter). This can be necessary during childbirth, in cases of renal colic, neurological pain and when ear acupuncture is used as an anaesthetic for operations. In such cases the needles may be inserted a little longer than would otherwise be customary, sometimes for several hours.

How long should the needles stay in?

Let the needles stay in place for at least 25, but preferably 40 minutes. In cases of severe pain it is better for the needles to stay in longer, for several hours.

Make sure that the patient is comfortable and relaxed during treatment, whether seated or lying down. Hopefully the patient will achieve a meditative state. Offer a blanket if it is cold in the room. Stay close by so you can hear if the patient calls. If there is no electrical alarm system in the clinic, the patient may feel more secure with a bell, or something similar, within easy reach to attract attention.

If the needles fall out

If one or several of the needles fall out directly after they have been inserted, a new, sterile needle can be placed in the point. If a needle falls out when more than half the treatment time has passed, there is no need to replace it.

Removing the needles

Removal of the needles when treatment is over does not usually cause the patient any discomfort.

It doesn't matter in which order they are removed. Take them out with a gentle movement and throw them immediately into a container for dangerous waste.

Have a cotton bud in your hand when you draw out the needles so you can quickly dry up any droplets of blood. Press for a few seconds against the point if it continues to bleed. (That is if bleeding technique is not being used (see further on in this chapter). If it *is* then of course the idea is that some drops of blood should run out.)

The blood-stained cotton buds should also be disposed of as dangerous waste.

Treating with semi-permanent needles

The great advantage of semi-permanent needles is that they give continual stimulation to a point for several days. Also they are simpler and cheaper for patients because they don't need to visit the acupuncturist as often. If semi-permanent needles are used, treatment time at the acupuncturist's is cut because the patient has no need to sit or lie with the needles inserted but can leave the clinic as soon as the needles are in place. The disadvantage is a slight increase in the risk of infection. The use of semi-permanent needles depends upon the patient being sober and able to react adequately to signs of infection. Semi-permanent needles are not usually used in NADA treatment (ear acupuncture used to treat addiction, see Ch. 13).

On the antihelix, on the helix root and at other places where needles are inserted into cartilage, semi-permanent needles are more painful. It can be better to use regular needles or pellets at such points in protruding parts of the ear.

Technique for semi-permanent needles

If semi-permanent needles are to be used it is doubly important for the ear to be clean because the needle will stay put and the risk of infection is therefore increased. When you have located points with your probe or electrical point detector, you'll see them as small indentations. Wipe them once more with alcohol and let them dry. The alcohol must have evaporated before you insert the needles in order to avoid it stinging. Then in peace and quiet insert the needle exactly into the little indentation left by the probe.

Press tacks

The use of semi-permanent needles in the form of press tacks requires greater dexterity of the fingers than when using ASP (acupuncture semi-permanent) needles. The simplest method is to lift the tack and its band aid to the point with the help of a pair of tweezers, making sure that the tip of the tack stays sterile. Then manoeuvre the tack using the tweezers so that the tip is right over the point. If the band aid to which the tack is attached is transparent, it will be easier to get this exactly right. When the band aid and the tack are in the right position, the ear acupuncturist pushes down on the band aid with index finger or pressure pen so that the tack goes through the skin and the band aid sits tight. At the same time the tweezers are taken away. (As an alternative to tweezers, the handle of a regular, sterile acupuncture needle can be used.)

Inform the patient how long the tack is to stay in place and how to remove it, also inform him of the risk of infection and what to do if the point should become infected (see page 157).

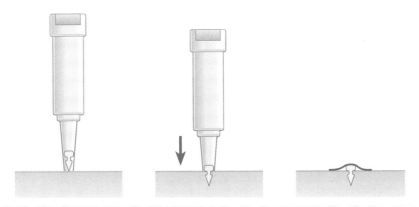

Figure 11.1 An ASP (acupuncture semi-permanent) needle in a tube pressed against the skin so that the needle is propelled into it.

ASP-type needles (see Fig. 11.1)

Hold the tube against the point chosen for treatment, which has been marked and wiped with alcohol. Make sure that the tip of the needle is right over the marked indentation. Pinch the ear with your free hand, ask the patient to take a deep breath, then firmly press the tube against the ear as the patient exhales. The tube is divided in the middle, so that one part slides into the other and the needle shoots out of it and into the skin.

Cover the needle with the round piece of skin-coloured band aid packed with the needle. This keeps the needle in place and protects the insertion point.

An ASP needle is thicker than a regular acupuncture needle, and than a press tack, and its insertion will be felt more keenly. But in compensation for this it will as a rule stay put longer. For the acupuncturist it is convenient and easy to place exactly where you want it.

If you send the patient home with the empty tube the needle can be stimulated now and then by the patient with the magnet which is attached to the other end of the tube. This possibly increases the effectiveness of the needle (though at the same time the risk of infection might also increase).

Inform the patient as to the length of time the tack must stay in place and how to remove it, also inform him of the risk of infection and what to do if the point should become infected (see page 157).

How long should a semi-permanent needle stay in place?

The effect of semi-permanent needles is more long term than that of regular needles. They will often fall out after about a week. They should not stay in place longer than 10 days. It is important to inform the patient of this and to demonstrate how they are to be removed.

Removing semi-permanent needles

ASP: remove the band aid. The needle will most likely come away with it. If not, carefully remove it with a clean pair of tweezers. Clean with alcohol and inspect the insertion point.

Press tack: when the band aid is removed with a clean pair of tweezers, the tack will come away with it because they are one unit. Clean with alcohol and inspect the insertion point.

Throw the needles immediately into a container for dangerous waste.

Risk of infection

The risk of infection is, as already mentioned, somewhat greater with the use of semi-permanent needles. Bearing in mind how many semi-permanent needles are used worldwide every day it is still minimal. This doesn't make it any the less unpleasant should an infection occur. The worst-case scenario is that this will be a cartilage infection, which can be difficult to cure. For this reason you should use semi-permanent needles with the greatest respect.

It is important to explain properly to the patient when and how to remove the needles and to keep the ear clean at the least sign of infection. If there is a reddening of the skin, a pulsating feeling or pain, the needles should be removed immediately. The ear should then be cleaned several times a day with soap and water or with alcohol. Tell the patient to come back so you can inspect the ear if any signs of infection. And if an infection should occur, the patient must be told to consult a doctor.

(In Chinese texts it is recommended that needles should be placed in the points External Ear, Kidney, Adrenal Gland and Brain if infection occurs.)

Semi-permanent needles should be used with greater care in warm climates, or when the patient is a keen swimmer or engaged in activities generating sweat, or when the risk of infection is increased.

Because of the risk of infection if the ear is not kept clean, semi-permanent needles are used only if the acupuncturist is sure that the patient is going to abstain from drugs or alcohol, and is able to judge if there are any signs of infection. If there are signs of infection the patient must have the ability to take out the needles, wash often with soap and water or with alcohol and seek the help of a doctor. This is why semi-permanent needles are seldom used during NADA treatment or in treating patients with psychiatric problems.

Does it hurt?

The moment of insertion of semi-permanent needles can be more painful than that of regular acupuncture needles. For hours afterwards the patient may be aware of the semi-permanent needles. This is normal. But if the needles start to cause pain after a few days, one should begin to suspect infection. Take out the needles immediately if there are any signs of infection.

If the patient says that it is painful to sleep with semi-permanent needles, put them in just one ear and if possible choose the ear which is not 'slept on'.

The number of needles

In treatment with regular acupuncture needles a maximum of five needles per ear is recommended.[4]

If you use semi-permanent needles, don't use more than six needles altogether in both ears.

---

[4] In NADA treatment (ear acupuncture for addiction, see Ch. 13) ten needles are used, five in each ear. As many needles are rarely used in other forms of ear acupuncture treatment.

Intervals between treatment

In cases of acute trouble and severe pain being treated with regular acupuncture needles one to three sessions a week may be necessary. With some conditions still more frequent treatment might be advantageous. Acute diarrhoea can, for example, be treated with two- to four-hour intervals between sessions.

As the problem diminishes, so the intervals between treatment can become longer, until the point is reached when the symptoms disappear and no treatment at all is necessary. If the symptoms return, of course, there may have to be a new course of treatment.

Chronic troubles and milder forms of pain can be treated sparsely, perhaps once a week or once a month.

In China treatments are more frequent than we are used to in the West, every day or every other day for 7–10 days. After that there's a week's pause before an equally intensive period of treatment begins.

Sicknesses in which there are periods of high and low activity are treated more frequently when the symptoms are most intense.

Treatment with semi-permanent needles can be given less frequently than that in which regular needles are used. In the beginning meet the patient every week or every other week, every week if you are uncertain and the patient feels insecure. When you are more confident and the patient feels more secure, it can be enough to meet the patient for back-up treatment every other month.

The amount of treatment differs according to each individual case. Around 5–10 treatments for acute injuries and 10–20 for chronic troubles can be necessary.

If the patient's condition hasn't improved after five to six treatments, change points. Consider whether there might be a therapy blockage (see page 167) which must be eliminated.

How to use pellets

The use of pellets or seeds (for the sake of simplicity, I shall in future refer to both as 'pellets') can be an alternative or a complement to treatment with acupuncture needles.

Find the active points to be treated. Wipe the ear with an alcohol swab so that the band aid will fasten properly. Tweezers can be a great help in putting pellets in place. (If you don't have tweezers, you can use a probe or the handle of a clean acupuncture needle.) Lift part of the band aid and pull it free from its packaging, manoeuvring it into the right position so that the pellet/seed is positioned right over the point to be treated. It'll be easier if the band aid is transparent. Push down on the band aid with the index finger of your free hand and take away the tweezers. Make sure that the pellet is in the correct position, right over the point you have chosen.

In principle, all points in the ear can be treated with pellets but putting a pellet in place on Sympathetic Autonomic Point and other points under the edge of the helix requires practice and dexterity with your fingers. Other aids may be necessary (for example an extra probe) if the point to be treated is in a place that is difficult to get to.

For increased effect, the patient can stimulate the point a few times a day by pressing down on the pellet (30 seconds' pressure — pause — 30 seconds' pressure).

The pellet can stay in place for several days, sometimes weeks. When the pellet has been in place for a few days it often forms a small indentation at the point. If the band aid is of good quality, one can shower and wash the hair without the pellet falling off. If the skin reddens or becomes irritated, the pellet should be taken away immediately.

When the pellet has been removed, you can put a new one in the same point providing that the skin has not reddened or become irritated.

Other methods of stimulation

Massage

It can be a good idea to massage the ear. We should begin with softly massaging the ears of our babies and continue the practice as they grow older. Young people and adults can quite easily learn to massage their ears themselves. Massaging the ear so that all the zones are stimulated can be a quick and simple way of giving yourself a body massage.

Massaging the ear:

Hold the ear so that the thumb massages the rear of the ear and the index finger the front.

1. Draw the ear upwards several times.
2. Then take the lobe and draw it downwards so that the ear is stretched out.
3. Hold the edge of the helix and draw the fingers up and down several times.
4. Hold and massage the lobe with circular movements.
5. Massage the edge of the antihelix…
6. …and then the bottom of the concha, using a circular motion of the index finger.
7. Take hold of the tragus and massage it several times using circular movements.

Finish up by rubbing the ear with the flat of your hand.
Feel how a pleasant warmth starts to spread.

You can systematically massage certain parts of the ear or specific points. It can be good for patients to learn how to treat their own symptoms. Show patients which zones are active and explain that it can be good if they give extra stimulation in these zones.

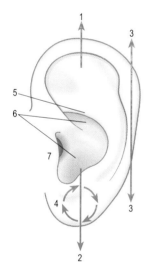

Figure 11.2 How to massage the ear.

Acupressure

Pressing a point with a probe is also a form of massage. The stimulation of specific points in this way is known as acupressure (a form of treatment in which one massages the acupuncture points instead of inserting needles in them). Often a glass probe with a thicker tip is used.

Most often the ear is palpated as a part of the examination. By letting your point detector linger on the active point a moment, you create a good preliminary to treatment, or a form of treatment itself. If treatment with acupuncture needles is inappropriate, for example because the patient is afraid of them, because there is danger of infection, or because the patient is too young, acupressure can be a valid alternative. If so, press for a few minutes on each active point.

When the active point is massaged with a probe, pain will initially increase. Continue the massage until the pain starts to diminish. This should take about one minute. According to Ralph Nogier, massaging the point in this way can have a surprisingly strong effect and may even cause fainting. He recommends that the patient should remain lying down and rest for half an hour after acupressure treatment.

If, after providing acupressure, you are going to treat with acupuncture, the probe will have left behind a small indentation at the active point, making it easier to see where the needles should be inserted.

Electrical stimulation

Electrical stimulation of the point may be administered in several ways. Either you insert regular acupuncture needles and connect them via small alligator clips to a TENS (transcutaneous electrical stimulation) apparatus (see Ch. 9, Equipment). In ear acupuncture two needles at the most are used for electrical stimulation in either ear. The acupuncturist chooses the frequency (Hz) and then slowly increases the intensity until the patient can tolerate no more. The treatment normally lasts 30–40 minutes. Electrical acupuncture in the ear can strengthen the pain-relieving effect and can be used, for example, during childbirth or surgery.

Another way to treat an ear acupuncture point with an electrical current is to use an advanced electrical point detector (see Ch. 9, Equipment) which can also be used to treat the point. When you have found the point it can be treated by pressing down the therapy button so that a weak stream of current is sent out via the probe. Using this type of electrical treatment, you can treat each point for about a minute, once or twice a week.

If you are using an AcuStim apparatus (see Ch. 9, Equipment), small paper electrodes are fixed to the points needing treatment. Thin cables are attached to the electrodes from the battery-driven AcuStim box. Patients can then turn the unit on and off, according to their needs or at regular intervals (for example a quarter of an hour each morning or evening). The patient can move during treatment. AcuStim can be used, for example, in treating pain or as an aid to slimming.

It can be a good idea to treat the points in the ear without inserting needles when patients are afraid of needles, have haemophilia, are carrying a blood-borne infectious disease or are too young to receive acupuncture proper.

Magnetic influence

Some researchers think that magnetic fields influence points in the ear, which is why some of the pellets marketed nowadays are magnetic.

ASP needles, the semi-permanent needles which are driven in with the help of the tube in which they are packed, can — during the period in which the needles stay in the ear — be stimulated with a small magnet to be found at the end of the tube. When the needle is in place, the empty tube can be given to the patient to take home. The patient can be instructed to hold the magnet against the needle several times a day. The aim is to make treatment more effective. (The disadvantage in instructing the patient to stimulate the needle is that the needle can be dislodged and that bacteria can easily find its way into the point.)

Heating with moxa

Moxa is used in body acupuncture according to traditional Chinese medicine (see Ch. 2, A brief look at traditional Chinese medicine (TCM)) to treat so-called 'cold' illnesses, for example rheumatic pain made worse by cold weather. A TCM acupuncturist can also choose to warm the zones in the ear which are pale, thought to be points corresponding to chronic damage or organs needing to be strengthened. Treating with moxa in the ear requires a steady hand and dexterity. The needles are short and are inserted only to a depth of a few millimetres making it impossible to fix a bit of a moxa stick to the needle, which is common in body acupuncture. It is risky to have glowing hot moxa so close to the hair and it is easy to burn the patient. It is impossible to warm a single point or a specific zone in the ear because the glowing moxa is too large and the points are too close together. However, if you still want to warm a point in the ear, you can use a moxa stick held above the needle. This should be adequately hot but not burn the skin. A treatment of three to five minutes should be enough.

Instead of burning moxa, the ear acupuncturist may warm the shaft of the needle with the flame of a cigarette lighter. It is difficult to regulate the warmth and there is a risk of burning the patient or setting fire to his hair.

An alternative to ordinary moxa in ear acupuncture is the use of a so-called 'tiger warmer' (a thin stick of moxa blended with other herbs) or an ordinary incense stick, both of which are considerably thinner than a regular moxa stick. They give, like regular moxa, an intensive warmth to the point but warm a smaller zone than a regular moxa stick, which is desirable when treating the ear.

Burning the ear

Formerly it was common to burn active points, particularly when treating sciatica and tooth ache. Madame Barrin, who showed Nogier how a zone in the ear could be burned when treating sciatica, used a small, flat piece of metal in which an oval hole had been made. She held the piece of metal so that the hole was over the zone she wanted to treat and pushed a piece of red hot metal against the hole. In this way a little oval burn sore formed in the ear.

Some of today's ear acupuncturists will take instead a metal paper clip, bend it out straight then hold it with a pair of tweezers in a flame until the tip is red hot. Then they press the red hot tip quickly against the desired point in the ear.

Bleeding the point

Bleeding, the release of a few drops of blood from an active point, is also known as microphlebotomy. First the ear is massaged to increase the flow of blood. With a triangular needle, a regular needle with a diameter of 0.30–0.90 mm or a lancet of the type used in taking fingertip blood samples, a point is pricked releasing one to five drops of blood. One can also make a small incision over the point with a larger scalpel and allow it to bleed for several minutes. The points which are most often treated in this way are Apex, Allergy, Urticaria Groove and Blood Pressure Groove on the rear of the ear. Two to four points can be bled in one session and the treatment may be repeated every three to five days if the point is pricked, or seven to ten days if the 'cutting method' (using the larger scalpel) is used. Three such treatments would normally be considered to be enough.

Bleeding technique is referred to in ancient Chinese texts. The method can be used in treating some acute inflammatory conditions, eczema and high blood pressure. It is also recommended for some chronic and difficult conditions. Nowadays the blood-letting method is less common.

After acute damage a dilated blood vessel can appear in the part of the ear corresponding to the injured body part. If, for example, a knee is injured during sporting activities, a red line may appear in the zone in the ear reflecting the knee. This may be interpreted as 'stagnation of blood' in TCM. If you insert a needle here so that there is a small amount of bleeding, the symptom may quickly disappear.

Inserting several needles in the same point

To increase the stimulation of a point, you can insert two or three needles into it simultaneously (see Fig. 11.3).

Injection therapy

A point in the ear may be treated by injecting different substances into it (0.1–0.3 ml). A small amount of anaesthetic, vitamin or antibiotic can be injected so that a small welt is formed, for example in the reflex point corresponding to the painful part of the locomotor system.[5] The injection into the point is repeated every two to three days.

Injection therapy is seldom used.

Stitches, staples and ear clamps

Nogier described in the 1980s how his colleagues would insert stitches (place threads) under the skin in the ear as an aid to get a patient to stop smoking. It was thought to give a more long-lasting effect than regular acupuncture needles but functioned with less precision than semi-permanent needles.

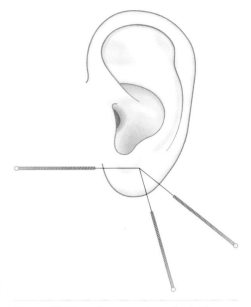

Figure 11.3 Inserting several needles in the same point.

Staples and ear clamps are thicker semi-permanent needles, shot into the ear with a device developed by a Russian scientist so that two points are connected to each other and remain attached for several days. The method was used in the 1970s as an alternative treatment for drug addicts.

These methods, which are not used for treatment nowadays, are reminiscent of piercing, in which a piece of metal is inserted through part of the body and fastened at each end with a metal stud.

Laser

In addition to inserting needles, burning or pressing points, they can also be radiated with a laser beam. Nogier has worked out a programme for laser treatment of the various zones of the ear. The point is irradiated for around 30 seconds. Laser treatment plays no part in the simpler form of ear acupuncture, or *auriculotherapy*, dealt with in this manual, but is used in *auriculomedicine*, which is beyond the scope of this book.

What can be treated with ear acupuncture

Ear acupuncture can have a relieving or supportive effect in the treatment of many different conditions. Pains, functional disturbance in, for example, the stomach and intestinal system or the urinary tract, allergies, dependence on alcohol, narcotics, nicotine or other substances, psychological symptoms, obesity, hormonal disturbances and

---

[5] The research team from Nanking suggested too that extracts of placenta and liver, and serum could be injected in the case of illnesses such as TB, asthma and infections. The method was also recommended as anaesthetic (Huang 1974).

some inflammatory illnesses and skin problems — all these are examples of symptoms that can respond well to ear acupuncture. (See Ch. 12, Treatment suggestions.)

A precondition is that the patient seeks help of his or her own free will, and has been examined by a doctor who has ruled out diagnosis requiring another form of treatment.

What can't be treated with ear acupuncture

- Congenital faults
- Major mechanical defects
- Cancer
- Degenerative diseases
- Diabetes.

(However, pain, anxiety and other symptoms in patients with such conditions can be alleviated by ear acupuncture.)

Contraindications, precautions

Contraindications fall into two categories, absolute and relative.

Absolute contraindications

- A life-threatening condition that requires another form of treatment.
- A condition that needs to be further investigated.
- Pains of indeterminate origin which can mean that another treatment (for example an operation) is necessary.
- Serious heart problems, patients who have had heart valve replacement surgery.
- Infected skin in the ear. On patients with eczema in the ear, external otitis or psoriasis one should not insert needles into the affected area. Use the active points that are located in healthy skin.

Relative contraindications

- Frostbitten ears.
- Ears with scars. Cauliflower ears (ears with a deformation after trauma) and ears that have undergone plastic surgery can react differently to acupuncture than unharmed ears.
- Intoxicated persons (unless it is the addiction that is to be treated).

■ *Continued*

- Patients who have been tortured or subjected to similar abuse can suffer frightening associations when undergoing acupuncture. Be extra careful and don't leave them alone during treatment.
- Patients taking anticoagulants (medicine that thins the blood) suffer increased bleeding risk.
- Patients with haemophilia. Consult with their doctor.
- For your own sake be extra careful with patients carrying infectious diseases such as HIV and hepatitis C.
- People with serious psychological disturbances who are not undergoing psychiatric treatment or who may be seeking acupuncture treatment that does not correspond with the psychiatric treatment they are being given.
- Allergies to the metal contained in the needles.
- Pregnant women, seriously ill patients and children (see below).

Pregnancy

Pregnancy is a relative rather than an absolute contraindication. Be especially careful when treating pregnant women. Remember you are treating both mother and foetus. There are points that influence the tone of the uterus and which should therefore be avoided during pregnancy. Use the points Uterus, Ovary and Endocrine with great care (or not at all) when treating pregnant women.

The points which are used in NADA treatment (Sympathetic Autonomic Point, Shen Men, Kidney, Lung and Liver) can be used during the entire pregnancy.

NADA treatment has been given to tens of thousands of pregnant drug abusers during all phases of pregnancy without side effects or causing harm to the foetus. On the contrary, it has been shown that pregnant women with a drug problem who are given ear acupuncture have a greater possibility of staying 'clean' during pregnancy. They carry their babies longer and there are fewer premature births. During treatment of cocaine users in the USA, children whose mothers were given ear acupuncture during pregnancy weighed nearly a kilo more at birth than those born to drug abusers who were not given ear acupuncture. NADA treatment has also allowed more children to be born without withdrawal symptoms.

Seriously ill patients

Ear acupuncture is powerful but no miracle worker. If you treat aged or weak patients, make sure they rest after the session. Patients who have fasted, who are anorexic or who haven't eaten properly for some other reason can have a stronger reaction against acupuncture. Be careful, insert fewer needles, let such patients lie down during treatment and stay in the room with them afterwards.

Children

The acupuncturist should see a child not as a small adult but rather as a being which functions in a completely different way. The meridians and points are not usually defined on small children. No scientific studies are available concerning ear acupuncture on children so we have no research to fall back on. Some countries have special rules concerning treatment of children. All acupuncturists should, of course, exercise extreme care in dealing with children.

Should treatment need to be given, my advice would be to treat a child with acupressure, pellets, electrical stimulation or laser treatment on active points, rather than with needles.

Expected reactions to treatment

Patients may experience a feeling of warmth in the ear, or that the ear has 'gone to sleep' or has grown larger. The ear may redden. The body can feel warm and relaxed. Sometimes sensations will be felt in the part of the body being treated. Pain can cease almost instantaneously.

A pleasant drowsiness or a great feeling of relaxation after treatment are common.

There may be an initial deterioration in the patient's condition a few hours or days after the treatment. Eczema may, for example, become more acute. Usually, this is a positive sign and the condition soon begins to get better.

Negative side effects

Infections

One negative side effect that has been reported after ear acupuncture is infection. The contagion may spread to other patients if the acupuncture needles are of a type that may be used several times and if sterilisation is faulty. It is for this reason that nowadays such needles are rarely used. It is a good idea to inform your patients that you are using disposable needles and that they need not worry about infection.

The risk of infection is greater if semi-permanent needles are used. For this reason special attention should be paid to hygiene during such treatment. Patients should also be carefully informed as to what they should do if signs of infection occur: 'If you experience pain around the semi-permanent needles, or pulsations and throbbing, or if the area becomes red and looks as if it is infected, you must remove the needles immediately. Keep the area clean using soap and water or by swabbing with alcohol several times a day. See your doctor if the irritation persists. Treatment with antibiotics may be necessary'.

Fainting

Patients may experience dryness in the mouth and feel dizzy as a result of acupuncture treatment. Sensitive persons may even faint. Fainting during body acupuncture treatment is uncommon, and is even less common during ear acupuncture. Be extra careful with patients who know they are sensitive, patients who haven't eaten for a long time, those who are afraid of acupuncture and with those who have a history of fainting when blood samples have been taken from them or they have been given injections. Insert only one or very few needles in such persons, making sure they lie down during treatment. Stay in the room with them.

If a patient faints: lay him/her down — if he/she is not already lying down — lift the legs, remove the needles and, above all, stay calm.

Bleeding

A small drop of blood can sometimes be seen when the needle is removed. Clean it away with a cotton bud. Press the bud against the point for a few seconds if a new drop appears or if there is more serious bleeding. It is most unusual that there will be any greater loss of blood than one or two drops. Inform the patient that this isn't dangerous, press with a cotton bud a few seconds more and keep calm. Take care not to expose yourself to blood-borne diseases, and avoid getting blood on your fingers.

(When using bleeding technique, the idea is that there should be blood. A thicker needle is used to extract a few drops of blood. See page 161.)

Positive side effects

Better sleep, improvement in mood and fewer worries are common side effects even when purely somatic troubles are being treated. This can lead to a cut back in consumption of tranquillisers and sleeping tablets.

It is also common that patients who suffer from premenstrual syndrome (PMS), headaches or irritable bowel syndrome report that such troubles diminish during the course of the treatment, even if these symptoms are not being treated specifically.

Another example of a positive side effect is that when acupuncture is used as an anaesthetic during tooth extraction; the blood vessels do not dilate as they do when a chemical anaesthetic is administered. In this way acupuncture provides better defence against infection and improves healing of sores.

When treatment is not successful

If the treatment has no effect, this can be because the diagnosis was wrong, that the choice of points was wrong or that the acupuncturist was trying to treat a complaint which was not suited to ear acupuncture. This can also be because the patient is a non-responder, because a certain medicine is having an influence on the effect of the acupuncture, or on other forms of therapy blockage.

Non-responders

Some patients remain in general unaffected by acupuncture. They are known as non-responders. No one knows exactly how large a group of people this is. A figure of between 5 and 10 percent is usually given.

Medicine

Simultaneous treatment with certain medicines that have an effect on the central nervous system and the autonomous nervous system can block the effects of acupuncture. One example are so-called beta-blockers, used to treat disturbances in heart beat, high blood pressure, angina pectoris, as a prophylactic for migraine and other problems. In a Finnish study of 1200 patients who were treated for being overweight, those that were taking beta-blockers (as blood pressure medicine) lost less weight (Pennala & Pönttinen 1985). Another example is cortisone, which, when given in high doses (more than 5 mg per day), reduces the effects of acupuncture. Neuroleptic medicine, antidepressants and tranquillisers, used to treat psychoses, depression, anxiety, worry and other complaints can also reduce the effects of acupuncture. Benzodiazepines are thought to have a particularly disturbing effect on acupuncture results. However, despite this, it is possible to treat symptoms of withdrawal from benzodiazepines with ear acupuncture, which otherwise can be extremely difficult to cope with. In fact ear acupuncture is an excellent aid in phasing out benzodiazepines.

Therapy blockage

According to Raphael Nogier, there are several other so-called blocks to effective auriculotherapy. Short descriptions of these follow.

Problems with laterality

If the two halves of the brain don't cooperate as they should, a series of symptoms will arise (see Ch. 5, Explanatory models for acupuncture, page 51, Laterality). The patient will also be difficult to treat if there are problems with laterality. According to Nogier these should be dealt with before other ear acupuncture treatment is given.

Food hypersensitivity

According to Nogier, after problems with laterality, wrong diet is the principal cause of general illness. By this he means eating food to which the body reacts negatively, almost as it would to poison. We are not talking here about allergy to certain foodstuffs (for example allergy to nuts, which gives rise to specific, acute symptoms) but a more diffuse sensitivity which depends on the amount eaten. For example, a person can tolerate a small amount of milk in food while being unable to drink milk by the glass. In such cases, it can be extremely difficult to work out just what it is that starts a reaction. To complicate matters still further, there may also be cross-tolerance. A person may be able to eat tomatoes and wheat separately but be unable to eat pizza. Another may tolerate milk only when not eating wheat.

Food hypersensitivity is trying for several reasons: partly because of the symptoms themselves, partly because it is difficult to work out from the symptoms just what it is that the person cannot tolerate and partly because of the difficulties in coming up with a new diet.

According to Nogier, those foodstuffs which most often cause food intolerance are milk, sugar, citrus fruits, coffee, tea, wheat, wine, beef, eggs, cooking oil, chocolate, rice and pork — in that order.

Symptoms that can arise if the organism is overloaded with food which it cannot tolerate can be general: high or low blood pressure, migraine, eczema, asthma, tiredness, allergies, cramps and hair loss, among others. The stomach and intestines may also produce symptoms, such as pains, diarrhoea and/or constipation.

There is no point in trying to deal with symptoms produced by food if this food is not eliminated from the diet. One should test each suspected foodstuff in turn. If the patient continues to eat food to which he or she is hypersensitive, acupuncture treatment will be less effective.

First rib syndrome

If the patient experiences a subluxation, or partial dislocation of the joint between the first rib bone and the first thoracic vertebra, many symptoms can arise in the sympathetic and parasympathetic nervous systems and may include heart trouble, diarrhoea, migraine-type headaches, conjunctivitis, neural pain or asthmatic problems. A partial dislocation may occur when, in attempting to lift a heavy object, the first rib bone is pressed out of position, onto a nerve in the sympathetic trunk.

If the patient's problem is that the rib bone is pushing on a nerve, a likely treatment is to adjust the rib bone so that it returns to the correct position. A chiropractor or a naprapath may be able to help.

Scars

In TCM it is believed that scars on the body could hinder circulation of qi, energy, if the scar 'cuts off' a meridian (see Ch. 2, A brief look at traditional Chinese medicine). If the qi doesn't flow as it should, a series of different symptoms can arise, depending on which meridian has been broken. Worst are long scars which lie diagonally across the abdomen or thorax. In body acupuncture the area around the scar can be treated to increase the possibilities for the qi to flow freely.

Even some Western doctors believe that scars may disturb bodily functions and provoke pathological reflexes. Such theories claim that a scar may destroy the relationship between the skin and the magnetic field of the surrounding world. In *Auriculotherapy Part 2* Coutté & Zorn (1999) say scars can affect the nervous system's contact with the outside world. They describe the skin as 'a radar, a fantastic organ, the connection between the inner world and all the stimuli of the external world, particularly light and colours'. This sensitivity can be damaged by scarring, they say. According to auriculomedicine, such damage can give rise to symptoms such as high or low blood pressure, depression, allergies and migraine.

The scars that cause problems are most often those that are tender to the touch. The symptom of which the patient complains is most often related to the occasion when the scar was formed. ('I've had high blood pressure ever since I was operated on for a meniscus injury in the knee. I couldn't take the anaesthetic' or 'After a bike crash four years ago, I've suffered from the most dreadful migraine'.)

A keloid scar (an elevated, irregularly shaped scar, formed with excessive amounts of collagen) which is large, reddened and swollen is the kind of scar most likely to cause problems, but even a mark left by a vaccination can be troublesome.

If the patient has a scar on the ear (perhaps as a result of a knife wound, an accident or an operation) avoid giving acupuncture at points within the actual scar.

Dental problems

A poor root filling, an encapsulated infection, an extracted tooth, fillings containing metals which produce an electrical field; all these may prevent ear acupuncture from achieving results. The patient may have sought treatment for toothache, but just as likely for sinus trouble, facial neuralgia, pains in an arm or shoulder, atypical pains or a series of other symptoms. It is difficult to get a good result with ear acupuncture without first dealing with the dental problem.

Posture anomalies and squinting

According to Nogier's school of thought distortions in the spine and/or feet, in the bite and squinting can give rise to different symptoms which can't be treated using ear acupuncture until the root cause has been corrected.

Other reasons

Other factors can worsen a prognosis. It is difficult to cure someone who actually benefits from being ill, or has unresolved social, family or work-related problems.

People with symptoms that may help in the settlement of an insurance claim or compensation for a work injury will most likely be easier to treat when their cases are settled.

12

Treatment suggestions

In this chapter we'll discuss how to choose the points to be treated and make suggestions for the treatment of different symptoms.

How to choose the points to be treated

If there is the least doubt concerning the reason for the patient's symptoms, a doctor should be consulted to rule out diagnoses that might call for some other form of treatment. Ear acupuncture, like all forms of treatment, has its limits. However, if the patient's symptoms are suitable for treatment with ear acupuncture, different principles should be applied in choosing the points to be treated.

When the patient has described the history of the illness and the symptoms, the acupuncturist can start to get a feeling for the points that may be suitable for treatment. When the ear has been examined, the acupuncturist will also know which points are active. Now it is time to choose the points to be treated.

Broadly speaking, there are two categories of points. The first group is the reflex points, each one corresponding to a part of the body. Every muscle, every bone, every inner organ has a reflex point in the ear. The second group is the functional points, which, as their name implies, influence bodily functions (read more about reflex points in Ch. 7 and functional points in Ch. 8). Most ear acupuncture treatments involve both reflex and functional points. In the following pages, we'll take a comprehensive look at the principles involved in choosing a point for treatment. Points from one or more of these principles can be chosen in the same treatment.

During the treatment period, active points can become inactive. In such cases you should choose other active points for treatment.

Prioritising active points

A basic principle is to only treat active points.[1] The active points that you have found in your examination are always worth treating. You should not insert more than five needles in each ear. If there are more than five active points, you will have to choose which of them are sorest or cause strongest reaction from your point detector. By all means change the choice of points from one session to the next.

You shouldn't merely consult a point chart and insert the acupuncture needles without searching for active points. Think rather of the zones on the point map as areas where you can expect to find active points. Remember you are looking at a projection of the parts of the body, an area where in all likelihood the points are to be found. There are no points for certain illnesses, but rather points that presumably have a relationship to the sick body part or organ.

However, if — despite a careful examination — you find no active points in the applicable zone, do the next best thing: look on the map for the point which corresponds to the part of the body causing pain or pathology and treat it.

Choosing the active point for a body part or organ

This is the simplest principle when it comes to choosing a point to treat. You've interviewed your patient and know what seems to be wrong. You know which body part or organ is causing pain or is malfunctioning. Now look for an active point in the zone of the ear corresponding to the part of the body in need of treatment. If the patient has stomachache, you look for the Stomach point and for tennis elbow, you look for the Elbow point.

Choosing the point for a function

Choose the functional point that corresponds to the malfunctioning experienced by the patient. Functional points are those points which empirically, from experience, have shown themselves to have an effect on the malfunction after which they have been named.

Example: choose the point Endocrine for irregular menstruation, Asthma for asthmatic breathing problems, Hunger to treat an appetite that is too large, Constipation when the intestine fails to empty. The point Allergy is used to diagnose and treat allergies. In cases of severe pain, it is important to treat one or more of the points that can relieve this, for example Shen Men, Thalamus or Analgesic.

Other functional points have a marked effect on our state of mind. They should be included if the patient is suffering from worry or anxiety.

Choosing masterpoints

Oleson (1998) gave five functional points the designation 'primary masterpoints'. These are thought to have a particularly powerful effect and are often used. They are: Sympathetic Autonomic Point, Shen Men, Point Zero, Thalamus and Endocrine.

---

[1] In NADA treatment, a standardised form of ear acupuncture used in treating addiction, the acupuncturist does not look for active points. See Ch. 13, NADA – using ear acupuncture to fight addiction in the beginning.

Oleson called five other points 'secondary masterpoints'. They were also seen as having a powerful effect and these points too are frequently used. They are: Master Oscillation, Allergy, the V-point, Master Sensorial and Master Cerebral.[2]

Masterpoints are potent functional points and one or more masterpoints are included in nearly all treatment programmes. Choose the masterpoint that is most relevant after deciding on the reflex points and possibly other functional points.

Choosing between active points

During the examination you may find more active points than you reckoned with. If so they can be treated. These 'reactive' points may be sore during palpation or register on your point detector. They may look different from the surrounding area or feel like a grain of sand to the touch. Such points are always worth treating.[3]

Point Zero geometry, the radius system

When you treat body parts and organs in the ear, you can find 'support' points on the antihelix, in the scaphoid fossa and on the helix. These form a geometric pattern. Because Point Zero is the principal reference point, the system is known as 'Point Zero geometry'. It is also called the 'radius method' or the 'segmental therapy' system. It is used first and foremost for treating pain or dysfunction in the locomotor system and in cases of pain in a particular segment.

The radius system can also be used to describe where a particular point is located. The location of an active point which in the illustration lies at number 2 can be described thus: 'The point lies on the helix in a direct line on a radius from Point Zero across the reflex point for C7' (see Fig. 12.1).

The starting point for treatment using Point Zero geometry is Point Zero and an active point. The active point can be the reflex point for a vertebra or a part of the body. Imagine a line drawn between these points and look for more active points along it. Where the line crosses the scaphoid fossa, or in the vegetative groove which lies half-hidden under the edge of the helix there is often an active point that is worth treating. Active points are often to be found in the sympathetic trunk, on the helix and on the antihelix. All active points on this line are worth treating.

Example 1: The patient has a pain in the elbow. Imagine a line drawn between Point Zero, through Elbow, over the helix. If you find an active point where the line crosses the scaphoid fossa, nearly under the edge of the helix, in the vegetative groove, it is definitely worth treating it.

Example 2: Another patient is suffering with neck trouble. An active point is found in the vegetative groove, on a line that runs between Point Zero and the reflex point for the fifth cervical vertebra, C5. Look along the imaginary line and you will often find more active points (see Fig. 12.2). They are all well worth treating.

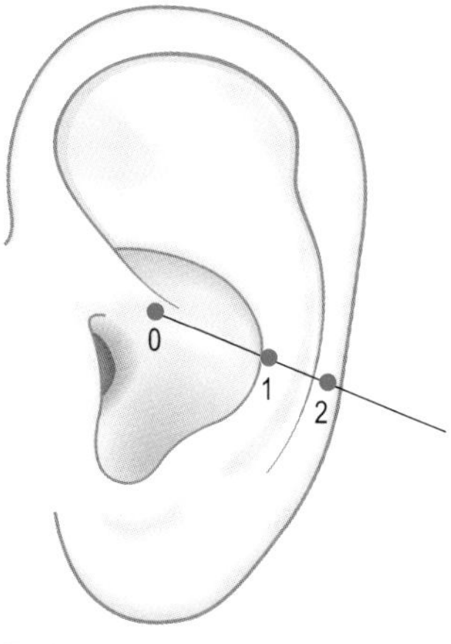

Figure 12.1 Point Zero geometry, the radius system.

0 = Point Zero
1 = Reflex point for C7
2 = Active point on the helix in a direct line on a radius running from Point Zero through the reflex point for C7

---

[2] In the third edition of Oleson's book (2003), he makes no distinction between primary and secondary masterpoints, simply calling them all 'masterpoints'.

[3] Nogier called the ear map described in this book 'phase one'. If you find reactive points in unexpected places, and study Nogier's 'four phases', you'll often find that these points are projected where the malfunctioning organ is listed, according to Phase Two or Phase Three. See page 174.

Choosing points in accord with TCM thinking on relationships

Those who have studied traditional Chinese medicine (TCM; see Ch. 2, A brief look at traditional Chinese medicine) will know that it attributes more and differing qualities to organs than those accorded to them by Western medicine and can use ear acupuncture according to these principles. The Chinese think that an energy disturbance in an organ and its meridian gives rise to registering of active points in the corresponding part of the ear. (This can explain the occurrence of some active points which on first examination appear to be illogical.) Using this theory, the points Spleen and Liver can be used, for example, to treat different bleeding disorders because, according to TCM, it is the spleen's job to keep the blood in place and the liver's is to store it and to see that it circulates freely.

Another example is that, according to TCM, each yin organ is manifested in a certain place in the body. According to this theory the liver 'opens' in the eye. Different eye troubles (dry eyes, bloodshot eyes, blurred vision, running eyes and other complaints) can, according to TCM, stem from disturbances in the functioning of the liver. For this reason Liver can be treated for most cases of eye trouble.

Similarly, because the lungs 'manifests' in the skin, the point Lung can be used to treat various skin complaints and because the kidney 'opens' in the ear, the point Kidney can be used to treat ear symptoms.

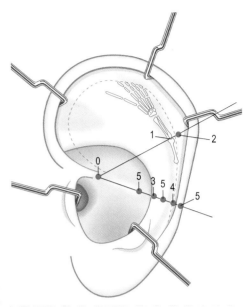

Figure 12.2 Point Zero geometry, radius lines.

0 = Point Zero
1 = Elbow
2 = Complementary point on the radial line
3 = Reflex point for cervical vertebra C5
4 = Active point in the vegetative groove
5 = Other active points along the radial line

Choosing the point for the paired organ using TCM

Those who have studied TCM can also choose points in the ear that are the equivalent of the affected organ's 'paired' organ. According to TCM, the organs' energy channels or meridians (energy channels in which the qi flows. See Ch. 2, A brief look at traditional Chinese medicine) are connected ('paired') in the following fashion: Lungs with Large Intestine, Stomach with Spleen, Heart with Small Intestine, Urinary Bladder with Kidney and Liver with Gallbladder. One can treat a complaint on the concerned meridian or via points on the meridian with which it is connected.

Example: the point Large Intestine can be used to treat asthma (because the large intestine's meridian is connected to the lungs) and skin troubles (because the lung opens in the skin). The point Spleen can be used to treat stomachache (the spleen's meridian is connected to the stomach's) and Small Intestine can be used to treat arrhythmias of the heart (the small intestine's meridian is connected to that of the heart).

Choosing the point for the meridian

Nogier didn't think that the meridians were represented in the ear but practitioners of Chinese ear acupuncture believe the opposite: that the meridians are reflected in the ear; and they choose points accordingly. To be able to treat illness according to this principle, you have to know how the meridians traverse the body. In this book we shan't go into the locations of the meridians but those who have studied Chinese medicine can try treating along the following lines.

If you are treating an injury in a part of the body with ear acupuncture and the treatment has not had the desired effect, then think about which meridian passes through the painful area and treat the point in the ear with the same name as the meridian.

Example: the patient has a pain in the knee. You have treated the points Knee (C) and Knee (F) without having an effect. Investigate which meridian passes through the part of the knee where the pain is located. If the pain is on the outside, where the gallbladder meridian passes, the Gallbladder point should be treated. If the rear of the knee is in pain, where the urinary bladder meridian passes, the Urinary Bladder point should be treated. If the pain is on the inside of the knee, where the spleen's meridian passes, treat instead the point Spleen.

Choosing points according to the Theory of the Five Elements

If you have been educated in TCM and know how the organs relate to the five elements, you can use the Theory of the Five Elements to choose points. In short the theory is based on a supposition that everything in the universe, in addition to being divided up into yin and yang, is also divided into the five elements (or phases): fire, earth, metal, water and wood. The internal organs too belong to one or other of these elements. In order for a person to be healthy, energy must circulate between the elements. The element that sends energy further is mother to the next element and at the same time son and receiver of energy from the element before it (see Fig. 12.3).

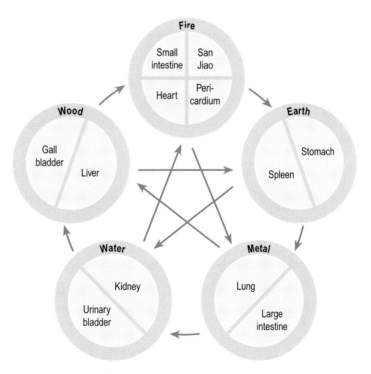

Figure 12.3 The organs' placing within the five elements. Yin organs lie towards the centre of the circle, yang organs furthest out.

If an organ is unbalanced, it can be treated in its own element. It can also be treated in the mother element (the element that lies before it in the circle) if the disturbance depends on the fact that the organ is receiving too little energy from the mother. A third alternative is to treat the troubled organ in the son element (the organ which comes after it in the circle) if the disturbance means that the son is drawing too much energy from the mother. A fourth alternative is to treat the organ in the element which lies two steps before it in the circle, if the disturbance depends on the fact that an organ in that element is not forwarding energy to its son, but is instead sending it forcefully past its son to the next element, with the result that the organs in that element are injured.

Example 1: if the problem, according to the TCM viewpoint, lies in a malfunctioning of the spleen, you can treat the Spleen point (its own element), the point Heart (the mother element), the point Lung (the son element), or the point Liver (the organ which lies two steps before in the circle).

Example 2: according to the Theory of the Five Elements, the point Kidney can be treated in cases of acute asthma (the kidney lies in the element water, which is son of the lung's element, metal). Kidney can also be used in cases involving anxiety which, according to TCM, is generated by 'fire in the heart' (Kidney, which lies in the element water, puts out fire which lies two steps onward in the circle).

Thinking in terms of Nogier's four phases

According to Nogier's phase theory there are three somatotopic systems on the front of the ear and one on the rear. According to this theory each body part can be represented at three different places on the front side of the ear and also on the back. Phase One is a projection of the body, which we have looked at in chapter 7. In Phase Two the backbone lies along the root of the helix, the large intestine on the tragus, arm and leg in the concha and the internal organs on the lobe. In Phase Three the spinal cord lies on the tragus, the intestines along the helix, the rest of the internal organs in the scaphoid fossa and on the antihelix and the arms and legs on the lobe.

If, after studying this book (Phase One), you don't understand why a certain point is reactive, it may prove rewarding to study Nogier's Phase Two and Phase Three. This can provide a solution as to why sometimes you cannot find an active point at the place it should be, and why you'll sometimes find active points in an unexpected place.

Phase Four is the back of the ear. There you'll find reflex points for many of the body's parts. They often lie directly opposite the point on the front of the ear. In this book we have looked at just a few of the points on the rear of the ear in Chs. 7 and 8, which describe reflex and functional points. By all means, also look for active points on the rear of the ear. If they are active, they too can be treated.

Suggestions for the choice of points, a point bank

In the remainder of this chapter, we'll look at the ear acupuncture points that can be treated for different symptoms. This will be a compilation of points suggested for treatment partly in the books I have used as a reference (see References), partly as a result of what I have learnt from different teachers. The choice is also characterised by personal experience. Look at them as a bank of possible points to be treated. There can be many reasons why a symptom arises. What caused a certain symptom in the patient you have in front of you can be decisive in choosing which points should be treated.

The point bank is not complete and the points are not arranged in order of importance. There may also be other points which in a special case are more suitable than those listed. Use the point bank for clues when looking for active points. Always give preference to the active points you find in examination. Choose the three to five most relevant points.

All the points in the point bank are described in Ch. 7, Reflex points, and in Ch. 8, Functional points.

Pain

Acute and chronic pain can be treated with ear acupuncture. It can, for example, ease pains in the musculature and skeleton, migraine and other headache, neurological pains (which in general are more difficult to treat), pains during and after childbirth, pain caused by surgical intervention and dental care.

Pain can be a warning signal. The acupuncturist should not take away symptoms which are a sign that another treatment is needed, so that the patient does not seek proper help. For example, pain in the abdomen should not be removed before its cause has been investigated. Before an acute athletic injury is treated, one should rule out a possible fracture or a dislocated joint. On the other hand, one can help patients suffering from toothache by relieving pain in the period when a patient is waiting for treatment by the dentist. A patient suffering pain from a newly operated knee can be given pain relief enabling him to commence physiotherapy and cut down on painkillers.

Pains in the locomotor system can be caused by poor posture, the adoption of an incorrect working posture and the lifting or carrying of loads in an incorrect way. In order for acupuncture treatment to have a lasting effect, it is important that the patient should perform exercises and adopt a correct working position. The patient may need help from a chiropractor, a naprapath, physiotherapist or an occupational therapist. If there is a psychological reason for the pain, this must be taken into account during treatment.

Point bank for pain

In my point bank Thalamus and Analgesic are the most potent points for relief of pain. Others that may have good effect are: Sympathetic Autonomic Point, Shen Men, Brain, Lesser Occipital Nerve and Neck. Hypothalamus is good for acute or chronic painful inflammation, Prostaglandin is excellent in cases of inflammatory pains in the joints. Master Cerebral lessens pain and anxiety. Muscle Relaxation and Jerome's Point can also be used in cases of pain because their treatment produces relaxation.

Point Zero is also included, partly because it can be used as a reference point in Point Zero geometry and partly because it has a general strong relaxing effect.

Adrenal Gland 1, Adrenal Gland 2, Kidney (C), Endocrine and Allergy are used if inflammation is a part of the pain problem. Vitality is also anti-inflammatory and is used during or after long illnesses.

Master Sensorial is used when the sensory stimuli are experienced as stronger than they are in reality. Urticaria Groove is recommended for shingles pain and Weather for aches and pains made worse by changes in the weather. Spleen is traditionally used in TCM to treat weak and painful musculature. Trigeminal Zone, Sciatica and Toothache are used for specific pain, as are the reflex points for the painful body part. Reflex points for the different parts of the body are described in Ch. 7.

See Figs. 12.4 and 12.5.

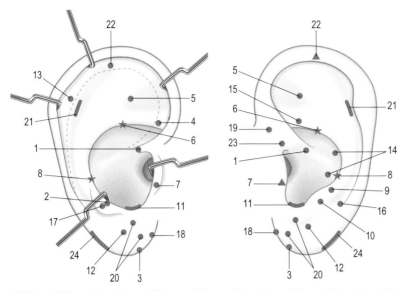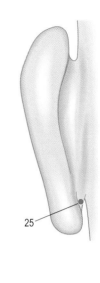

Figures 12.4 and 12.5 Point bank for pain.

1. Point Zero
2. Thalamus
3. Analgesic
4. Sympathetic Autonomic Point
5. Shen Men
6. Adrenal Gland 1

7. Adrenal Gland 2
8. Muscle Relaxation
9. Neck
10. Brain
11. Endocrine
12. Master Sensorial
13. Lesser Occipital Nerve

14. Spleen (F) and (C)
15. Sciatica
16. Jerome's Point
17. Hypothalamus
18. Master Cerebral
19. Weather
20. Toothache

21. Urticaria Groove
22. Allergy
23. Vitality
24. Trigeminal Zone
25. Prostaglandin

General advice for treating pain

Always look for an active point for the part of the body causing pain.

By all means use Point Zero geometry: imagine a line from Point Zero through the reflex point for the vertebra corresponding to the segment concerned, or through the reflex point for the painful body part. Look for active points in an extension of this line in the sympathetic trunk, vegetative groove, in the scaphoid fossa and on the helix. Treat the active points you find on this line.

Acute pain

Thalamus and Analgesic are points which are especially good in cases of intensive pain.

Pain in a joint, joint inflammation, tennis elbow, swollen joints, frozen shoulders

Point Zero geometry (see page 171). Reflex point for the painful body part. Endocrine, Kidney, Adrenal Gland 1 and 2, Shen Men, Prostaglandin, Point Zero, Muscle Relaxation, Neck, Lesser Occipital Nerve.

If there is a worsening with a change in the weather, treat the Weather point.

Muscular cramp

Reflex point for the painful body part. Point Zero, Thalamus, Spleen, Muscle Relaxation.

If there is a worsening with a change in the weather, treat the Weather point.

Backache/sciatica

Point Zero geometry, see page 171. Thalamus and Analgesic if pain is acute. Reflex points for the vertebrae and muscles involved (search both the zones for the discs, the vertebrae and the zone for the muscles at the part of antihelix facing the helix). Sciatica (firstly, on the side where the pain is located, eventually on both sides), Point Zero, Neck, Adrenal Gland 1 and 2, Jerome's Point, Muscle Relaxation, Hypothalamus, Shen Men, Sympathetic Autonomic Point, Master Omega.

Wryneck, whiplash

Point Zero geometry, see page 171. Thalamus and Analgesic if pain is acute. Reflex points for the vertebrae involved, Neck, Point Zero, Shen Men, Thalamus, Shoulder Blade, Collarbone, Jerome's Point, Muscle Relaxation, Sympathetic Autonomic Point, Hypothalamus, Master Omega.

Fibromyalgia

Point Zero geometry, see page 171. Reflex point for the body parts causing pain. Points which correspond to the vertebrae involved, Point Zero, Shen Men, Thalamus, Kidney (C), Neck, Jerome's Point.

If there is a worsening with a change in the weather, treat the Weather point.

Rheumatic pain

Point Zero geometry, see page 171. Reflex point for the body parts causing pain, Point Zero, Shen Men, Thalamus, Endocrine, Adrenal Gland 1 and 2, Kidney (C).

If there is a worsening with a change in the weather, treat the Weather point.

Phantom and stump pain

Point Zero geometry, see page 171. Thalamus and Analgesic if pain is acute, Shen Men, Forehead, Brain, points corresponding to the missing body part.

Shingles

Shingles (herpes zoster) is a virus outbreak which can give difficult and — in the case of older patients — prolonged neurological pain. Use Thalamus and Analgesic if the pain is acute. Point Zero geometry, see page 171. Look along the entire line leading from Point Zero through the reflex point for the vertebra where the nerve that is concerned issues from spinal cord. Look in the entire segment, in the vegetative groove, in the sympathetic trunk and in the zone for the spinal cord on the helix. Other points: Lung, Brain, Shen Men, Urticaria Groove, Allergy, Vitality, Adrenal Gland 1 and 2, Endocrine, reflex points for the part of the body concerned, Master Cerebral.

Pain after fracture

Point Zero geometry, see page 171. Thalamus and Analgesic if pain is acute. Reflex points for the corresponding part of the body. Kidney, Thalamus, Adrenal Gland 1 and 2, Shen Men.

Trigeminal neuralgia

Trigeminal neuralgia gives rise to brief but very intense attacks of pain in the area innervated by the trigeminal nerve. Point bank: Thalamus, Analgesic, Cheek, Jaw, Trigeminal zone, Brain, Liver, Mouth, Shen Men, Lesser Occipital Nerve. Look for active points in both ears.

Toothache

Thalamus and Analgesic if pain is acute. Jaw, Apex, Teeth.

Headache

Investigate all reasons and possible diagnoses for the headache. Headache can be a warning signal. Encourage the patient to see a doctor if the headache has suddenly come about, in cases of loss of speech, sight, movement or hearing, if the patient has cramps or has experienced a sudden change of personality.

There can be many reasons for headache. Stress, poor quality of indoor air, too little sleep, anxiety, medicine, addiction to medicaments (not least those obtainable without prescription), hunger, hypersensitivity to food (or 'triggers' such as red wine, alcohol, chocolate, chemical additives and sugar), too little exercise, dehydration, muscular tension, sight problems, sinus infection, tension in jaw bone joints, grinding together of teeth at night, constipation, too high or too low blood pressure, meningitis, concussion, tumour (primary or metastatic), stroke — all these are examples of conditions that can give rise to headache.

Discuss with the patient the possibility that a change of lifestyle might be needed to get rid of the headache. If the patient is out of sorts with his home or work environment, drinks too little (water) or too much (alcohol), acupuncture will have only a short-term effect, unless these and other headache-causing factors are cleared up. Other factors may help to keep headaches at bay, such as better posture, an improved working environment and a change of such habits as hunching the shoulder to hold a telephone, or carrying a shoulder bag always on the same side. Other patients need to learn how to relax, to say no, to cultivate better eating and sleeping habits or to stop taking painkillers for their headaches. Ironically, headache tablets can create withdrawal symptoms, which include headaches — a vicious circle in which the patient takes medicine to get rid of the withdrawal symptoms from the same medicine. A gradual reduction of medicine can be time-consuming but necessary and here ear acupuncture can be of great help.

Point bank for headache

See Fig. 12.6.

Migraine

During the attack: Thalamus, Analgesic, Allergy (bleeding technique), Shen Men, Brain, Point Zero, Neck, Point Zero geometry — look for active points on the imaginary lines that run from Point Zero through the cervical vertebrae.

Between attacks: Temple, Forehead, Brain, Shen Men, Sympathetic Autonomic Point, Hypothalamus, Point Zero, Neck, Master Cerebral, Frustration, Aggression, Jerome's Point, Lesser Occipital Nerve. Point Zero geometry: look for active points in the vegetative groove on an extended imaginary line between Point Zero and the

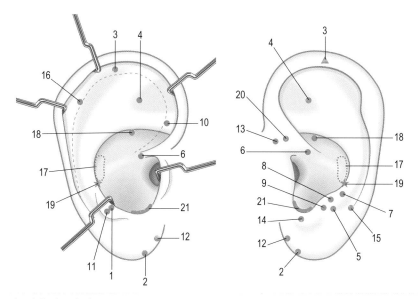

Figure 12.6 Point bank for headache.

1. Thalamus
2. Analgesic
3. Allergy
4. Shen Men
5. Brain
6. Point Zero
7. Neck
8. Temple
9. Forehead
10. Sympathetic Autonomic Point
11. Hypothalamus
12. Master Cerebral
13. Frustration
14. Aggression
15. Jerome's Point
16. Lesser Occipital Nerve
17. Liver
18. Kidney (C)
19. Muscle Relaxation
20. Weather
21. Endocrine

reflex points for the cervical vertebrae. According to TCM, Liver and Kidney can also be suitable points for treatment.

Tense headaches

Neck, Brain, Forehead, Temple, Shoulder Joint, Shoulder Blade, Shen Men, Thalamus, Hypothalamus, Muscle Relaxation, Jerome's Point, Master Cerebral.

If the headache is hormonal: Endocrine, Uterus, Ovary.

If the headache is connected with the weather: Weather.

If the headache gives rise to nausea and vomiting: Stomach, Point Zero, Neck.

Skin complaints

Point bank for skin complaints

See Fig. 12.7.

Begin with the reflex point for the part of the body affected. The points Skin Disorder and Urticaria Groove may be treated in the case of most skin symptoms. Add to these Allergy, Thymus, Endocrine and Adrenal Gland 1 and 2 in cases of

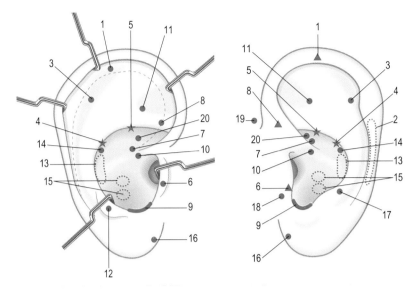

Figure 12.7 Point bank for skin complaints.

1	Allergy	7	Large Intestine	12	Hypothalamus	18	V-point
2	Skin Disorder	8	Sympathetic Autonomic	13	Liver	19	Psychosomatic
3	Urticaria Groove		Point	14	Gallbladder	20	Hypogastric Plexus
4	Thymus	9	Endocrine	15	Upper and Lower Lung		
5	Adrenal Gland 1	10	Point Zero	16	Master Cerebral		
6	Adrenal Gland 2	11	Shen Men	17	Neck		

allergic reaction and nettle rash. Shen Men has an antiallergic effect and Sympathetic Autonomic Point, Hypothalamus and Point Zero have a generally stabilising effect.

Add Liver and Gallbladder for skin troubles that crop up suddenly and then disappear. Use Hypogastric Plexus if the problem is accentuated after intake of food and Master Cerebral, Neck, the V-point and Psychosomatic if there are psychological factors to be taken into account.

According to TCM, the lungs open in the skin and the lung meridian is connected to that of the large intestine so the points Lung and Large Intestine are used in ear acupuncture for troubles that manifest themselves on the skin. According to TCM, kidney energy governs growth of hair and the point Kidney is used to treat early hair loss on the assumption that kidney energy must be weak.

Eczema, itching, nettle rash

First try to find the reasons for the outbreak of eczema and/or itching. It can be caused or made worse by a medicinal side effect, a contact allergy, an infection, a stress symptom or a reaction to something in the diet. Itching can arise without eczema and be a sign of dried-out skin, scabies, gall or liver sickness, uraemia, malignancy or psychosis. What may be needed are changes in diet or lifestyle, or the removal from the immediate environment of the substance causing the allergy.

Point bank: Allergy (use bleeding technique if the eczema is widespread), the reflex point for the part of the body concerned, Skin Disorder, Thymus, Adrenal Gland 1 and 2, Sympathetic Autonomic Point, Urticaria Groove, Endocrine, Point Zero, Shen Men, Hypothalamus, Liver, Gallbladder, Kidney. If the symptoms are increased by stress: Master Cerebral, Neck, the V-point and Psychosomatic. If the symptoms are made worse by something in the diet: Hypogastric Plexus. According to TCM: Large Intestine and Lung.

Acne

Skin Disorder and Urticaria Groove, Point Zero, Shen Men, Endocrine, the reflex point for the affected body part. According to TCM: Lung, Large Intestine.

Acne rosacea

External Nose (F) and (C), possibly with bleeding technique, Skin Disorder and Urticaria Groove, Lung, Shen Men, Endocrine, Adrenal Gland 1 and 2, Spleen, Apex.

Erysipelas

Can need treatment with antibiotics. Point bank: reflex point for the affected body part, Lung, Brain, Adrenal Gland 1 and 2, Endocrine.

Sunburn

Reflex point for the affected body part, Skin Disorder, Point Zero, Shen Men, Lung, Adrenal Gland 1 and 2.

Perspiration (in abnormally large amounts)

Sympathetic Autonomic Point, Lung, Endocrine, Brain, Thalamus, Hypothalamus, Point Zero, Adrenal Gland 1 and 2, Shen Men, reflex point for the affected body part, active points in the zone for the sympathetic trunk, Neck, Heart.

Hair loss

Kidney (C), Lung, Endocrine, Brain, Neck, Point Zero, Shen Men. If only in certain spots: Liver.

Scars

In treating disturbances that have arisen in the body because of scarring, Nogier recommends Point Zero geometry (see page 171). Treat the active points on the imaginary line from Point Zero through the reflex point for the scarred body part. Use regular or semi-permanent needles. If the scar is a long one (such as after bilateral plastic breast surgery), both ears are treated.

If the patient has a scar on the ear (perhaps as a result of a knife wound, an accident or an operation) avoid giving acupuncture at points within the actual scar.

Symptoms of heart and blood circulation troubles

Rule out serious heart disease which obviously needs other treatment.

Point bank for heart trouble

See Figs. 12.8 and 12.9.

Begin with Heart 1 and 2 (C), Heart (F) and Cardiac Plexus if they are active.

Apex is used in acute situations. Sympathetic Autonomic Point, Point Zero, Shen Men, Vagus Nerve, Endocrine, Hypothalamus and Thalamus help regulate the functioning of the heart. The point Blood Pressure and the Blood Pressure Groove

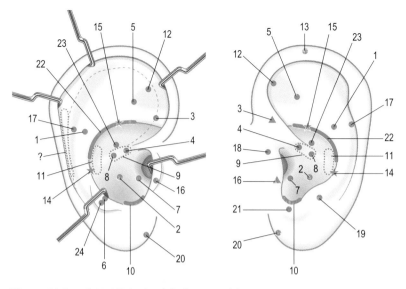
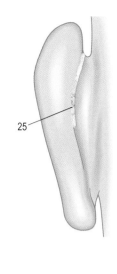

Figure 12.8 and 12.9 Point bank for heart trouble.

1. Heart (F)
2. Heart 1 (C)
3. Sympathetic Autonomic Point
4. Point Zero
5. Shen Men
6. Thalamus
7. Vagus Nerve
8. Stomach
9. Solar Plexus
10. Endocrine
11. Liver
12. Blood Pressure
13. Apex
14. Cardiac Plexus/Muscle Relaxation
15. Adrenal Gland 1
16. Adrenal Gland 2
17. Beta-1 Receptor Point
18. Heart 2 (C)
19. Brain
20. Master Cerebral
21. Aggression
22. Circulatory System
23. Small Intestine
24. Hypothalamus
25. Blood Pressure Groove

regulate both high and low blood pressure and Beta-1 Receptor Point help to lower blood pressure.

Adrenal Gland 1 and 2, Brain, Master Cerebral, Stomach, Solar Plexus, Aggression, Muscle Relaxation and other calming points can be a useful addition if stress has caused or worsened the symptom.

According to TCM, the heart's meridian is connected to that of the small intestine, and one of the liver's tasks is to see that everything circulates as it should. The spleen makes sure that liquid in the body is transported and transformed. For this reason the ear acupuncture points Small Intestine, Liver and Spleen are used in cases of heart and blood circulatory problems.

Angina pectoris

Heart 1 and 2 (C) and Heart (F), Sympathetic Autonomic Point, Point Zero, Shen Men, Thalamus, Vagus Nerve, Stomach, Solar Plexus.

Impaired blood circulation, cold hands and feet

Heart 1 and 2 (C) and Heart (F), Sympathetic Autonomic Point, Shen Men, Endocrine, Thalamus, Liver, reflex points for the part of the body affected.

High blood pressure

High blood pressure can be a serious health risk and should be thoroughly investigated. It can have many causes, including overweight, stress, kidney dysfunction, hormonal imbalance. Recommend exercise, a sound diet, weight loss if the patient is overweight, and recommend that the patient eliminates other factors which heighten the risk for heart and vascular illness, such as smoking. If the patient wishes to stop taking medicine for blood pressure, a gradual reduction should only be made in consultation with the doctor he is consulting.

Point bank: Blood Pressure, Shen Men, Sympathetic Autonomic Point, the Blood Pressure Groove on the rear of the ear, Apex (traditionally with bleeding technique), Cardiac Plexus, Heart 1 and 2 (C), Heart (F), Adrenal Gland 1 and 2, Liver, Neck, Thalamus, Hypothalamus, Brain, Master Cerebral, Aggression, Beta-1 Receptor Point, Vagus Nerve, Point Zero, Muscle Relaxation, Endocrine.

Low blood pressure

The same points are often recommended for this as for high blood pressure. (Acupuncture is a regulating treatment.) There is a point in the Endocrine Zone which in certain texts is known as Low Blood Pressure.

Palpitation, arrhythmias, bradycardia

Cardiac Plexus, Sympathetic Autonomic Point, Shen Men, Heart 1 and 2 (C), Heart (F), Master Cerebral, Thalamus, Vagus Nerve, Point Zero, Adrenal Gland 1 and 2. According to TCM, Small Intestine.

Raynaud's syndrome

Reflex points for the part of the body affected, Heart 1 and 2 (C), Heart (F), Sympathetic Autonomic Point, Endocrine, Adrenal Gland 1 and 2, Lesser Occipital Nerve, Shen Men, Thalamus, active points in the sympathetic trunk, Neck, Liver, Spleen.

Oedema, swelling

Kidney (C), Urinary Bladder, Heart 1 and 2 (C), Heart (F), Sympathetic Autonomic Point, Endocrine. According to TCM: Spleen and Liver.

The respiratory tract, and ear, nose and throat problems

Point bank

See Figs. 12.10 and 12.11.

Choose first active reflex points for the organs concerned, for example Lung, Bronchi, Trachea, Throat, Tonsils, Inner Nose, Forehead, Mouth, Palate, Cheek, Eye, Ear (there are three eye points and three ear points), Salivary Gland and Auditory Nerve.

Add Allergy, Asthma, Thymus and Adrenal Gland 1 and 2 if there is an allergic or inflammatory aspect to the problem.

Point Zero, Shen Men, Sympathetic Autonomic Point, Hypothalamus, Brain, Vagus Nerve and San Jiao are regulating. Lesser Occipital Nerve, Neck, Master Cerebral, Psychosomatic, Jerome's Point and other calming points may be used if there are psychological factors to be taken into account. Vitality may be added in cases when illness is long and drawn out and when immune defence is impaired, Weather when symptoms are accentuated by a change in the weather, Apex when

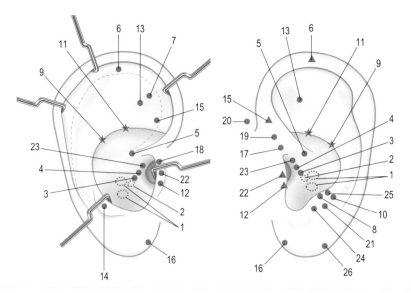

Figure 12.10 Point bank for illness in ear, nose, throat and respiratory tract.

1. Upper and lower lung
2. Bronchi/Bronchitis
3. Trachea
4. Throat (F)
5. Point Zero
6. Allergy/Apex
7. Asthma 1
8. Asthma 2
9. Thymus
10. Neck
11. Adrenal Gland 1
12. Adrenal Gland 2
13. Shen Men
14. Hypothalamus
15. Sympathetic Autonomic Point
16. Master Cerebral
17. Vitality
18. Throat (C)
19. Weather
20. Psychosomatic
21. Brain
22. Inner Nose
23. Mouth
24. Forehead
25. Cough
26. Sneeze

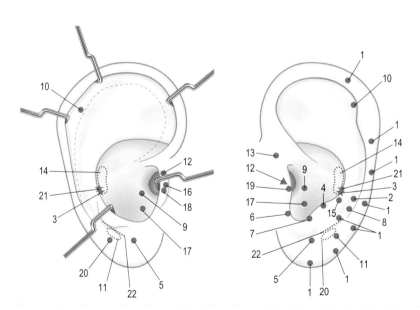

Figure 12.11 More points used to treat ear, nose and throat and respiratory illnesses.

1. Tonsils
2. Thyroid 1
3. Thyroid 2
4. Salivary Gland
5. Eye/Master Sensorial
6. Eye 1
7. Eye 2
8. Jerome's Point
9. Vagus Nerve
10. Lesser Occipital Nerve
11. Inner Ear (C)
12. Inner Ear (F)
13. External Ear
14. Liver
15. Cerebellum
16. Auditory Nerve
17. San Jiao
18. Master Oscillation
19. Thirst
20. Cheek
21. Muscle Relaxation
22. Auditory Zone

the situation is acute, Thirst if the mouth is dry, Cough and Sneeze as required, Master Oscillation if there is a problem with laterality, Thyroid 1 and 2 if there is a goitre or other throat symptom. Master Sensorial can be used when the sensory stimuli are experienced as being stronger than they are in reality.

According to TCM, the kidney 'opens' in the ear, the spleen is important for the immune defence system and stagnated liver energy can give rise to a feeling of having a lump in the throat ('plum stone sensation'). The meridian with the name San Jiao (Triple Heater) goes around the ear. This is why the ear points Kidney (C) and San Jiao are used to treat ear symptoms, Liver to treat the feeling of a lump in the throat and Spleen to boost the immune defence system in the case of recurring infection.

General thoughts on treating infections

Most infections of the respiratory tract are viral. In such cases antibiotics cannot help. Acute bacteriological infection, on the other hand, may require treatment with antibiotics. Ear acupuncture can stimulate immunity but has no antibiotic effect. If the patient is susceptible to infection, acupuncture may be used to stimulate immunity. If there is a latent infection which has a tendency to flare up when the patient is for some reason weakened, acupuncture can boost powers of resistance.

Asthma

Asthma is an illness that can be life-threatening. Acute attacks in which the patient is generally debilitated require treatment by a doctor. If the patient does not wish to continue to use prescribed medicine, it should be reduced only in consultation with the doctor who is treating the condition. Infections, smoky environments and other pollutants and allergenics can spark off an attack. Encourage patients who smoke to kick the habit.

Acute asthma attack: Allergy (use bleeding technique). Point Zero geometry: active points on the line that runs through Point Zero and Ganglion Stellatum. Thymus, Asthma 1 and 2, active points in the Lung Zone, Bronchi, Neck, Adrenal Gland 1 and 2, Shen Men, Sympathetic Autonomic Point, Point Zero, the V-point, Hypothalamus, Master Cerebral, Cough.

Between attacks: Allergy, Thymus, Trachea, Bronchi, Sympathetic Autonomic Point, Point Zero, Vitality, Kidney (C), Neck. Weather if the asthma attack is brought on by a certain form of weather. Master Cerebral, Spleen, Psychosomatic.

Bronchitis

Active points in the Lung Zone, Bronchi/Bronchitis, Trachea, Asthma 1 and 2, Sympathetic Autonomic Point, Point Zero, Shen Men, Allergy, Adrenal Gland 1 and 2, Neck.

Chronic bronchitis: Encourage patients who smoke to kick the habit. See if there might be the possibility of improving the quality of the air indoors both at home and work if it is of poor quality. Stimulate the immune defence system if it is impaired. Additional point: Vitality.

Cough, whooping cough

Asthma 1 and 2, Sympathetic Autonomic Point, Point Zero, Adrenal Gland 1 and 2, Bronchi, Brain, Lung, Shen Men, Neck, Cough.

Colds, influenza

Inner Nose, Throat, Forehead, Lung, Point Zero, Shen Men, Asthma, Allergy, Thalamus, Adrenal Gland 1 and 2, Spleen, Cough.

Hoarseness, sore throat

Trachea, Bronchi, Throat, Mouth, Tonsil points, Prostaglandin, Point Zero, Shen Men, Lung, Endocrine, Adrenal Gland 1 and 2.

Tonsillitis

Tonsillitis with a high temperature may require treatment with antibiotics. Point bank: Throat, Tonsil Points (many of them may be active), Trachea, Thyroid, Point Zero, Shen Men, Apex. Apex and the Tonsil Points can be treated with bleeding technique.

Sinusitis

Sinusitis can develop into therapy-resistant chronic recurrent infections. Point bank: Inner Nose, Forehead, Cheek, Point Zero, Shen Men, Asthma, Allergy, Lung, Adrenal Gland 1 and 2, Vitality.

Inflammation of the ear, otitis

Inner Ear (C) and Inner Ear (F), Kidney (C), Point Zero, Shen Men, Adrenal Gland 1 and 2, External Ear, Neck, San Jiao, Apex, Master Cerebral.

Mumps

Cheek, Salivary Gland, Endocrine, Thalamus.

Hay fever, allergic rhinitis

Preferably start treatment a month before the hay fever season starts so that the patient has had at least five sessions before the allergens start to affect them. Begin with more frequent treatment (twice a week), then gradually increase the time between sessions if you don't use semi-permanent needles. By the last half of the season, once every fourth week should be enough.

Acute phase: Inner Nose (C) and (F) when there is runny nose and sneezing, Allergy (use with bleeding technique), Adrenal Gland 1 and 2, Endocrine, Shen Men, Thymus, Eye, Eye 1 and Eye 2 if the eyes are irritated, active points in the zone for the sympathetic trunk close to the reflex points for cervical vertebrae C1–C7.

Latent phase: Choose between the active points mentioned above, plus Lung, Kidney (C), Vitality.

Goitre, over- and under-functioning thyroid

Thyroid 1 and 2, active points in the Endocrine Zone, Point Zero, Shen Men, Brain, Master Oscillation, Apex.

Feeling of a lump in the throat

Point Zero geometry: look along an imaginary line running from Point Zero through the reflex point for the throat, particularly in the vegetative groove. Throat, Larynx, Trachea, Sympathetic Autonomic Point. If there is psychological stress: Master Cerebral, Jerome's Point. According to TCM: Liver.

Difficulties in swallowing

Mouth, Throat, Vagus Nerve.

Dry mouth

Salivary Gland, Thirst, Mouth, Endocrine, Shen Men, Sympathetic Autonomic Point.

Nosebleed

Inner Nose, Forehead, Adrenal Gland, Lung, Apex.

Tinnitus

Tinnitus, a buzzing or ringing in the ears, is a common symptom which can have many causes: damage from working in noise or being in concert halls with too high sound level, tense muscles in the jaw and neck, infection, foreign bodies in the ears and even certain medicaments. Tinnitus can be extremely irritating for the person affected and is difficult to treat. Conventional healthcare seldom results in an effective cure. Muscular relaxation and adjustment of the patient's bite can sometimes lead to a reduction in the symptom. The problem is made worse by stress, tiredness, a large intake of coffee and depression. Music or some other background noise can lessen the awareness of tinnitus. Acupuncture can relieve the symptom or make it easier to withstand the experience of the buzzing in the ears.

Point bank: Inner Ear (C) and (F), External Ear, Point Zero, Shen Men, Cervical Vertebrae, Neck, Shoulder, Brain, Forehead, Auditory Zone, Sympathetic Autonomic Point, Hypothalamus, Master Cerebral, Master Sensorial, active points in the zone for the sympathetic trunk, Auditory Nerve, San Jiao, Master Oscillation, Adrenal Gland 1 and 2, Lesser Occipital Nerve, Muscle Relaxation, Jerome's Point. According to TCM: Liver and Kidney.

Ménière's disease

Sympathetic Autonomic Point, Hypothalamus, Auditory Zone, Neck (in or just above Neck there is a point which has an influence on nausea), Point Zero, Kidney, Shen Men, Brain, Cerebellum, Inner Ear, Thalamus, Lesser Occipital Nerve, Master Sensorial.

Eye problems

All patients with symptoms that can indicate a disease with a risk to eyesight must be sent to a doctor for examination and treatment.

Point bank for eye symptoms

See Fig. 12.12.

The eye has three reflex points. Use those which are active. In the case of recurring infections it may be a good idea to add Thymus, Vitality and Adrenal Gland 1 and 2. Skin Disorder and Urticaria Groove are also used to treat eye problems, as is Endocrine. Shen Men has an anti-allergic and anti-inflammatory effect. Apex is used in acute cases.

According to TCM, the liver 'opens' in the eye. Therefore the ear point Liver is used to treat eye symptoms.

Allergic conjunctivitis

When the eyes are irritated because of an allergy: Allergy (bleeding technique if the allergy is most acute), Eye, Eye 1 and 2, Thymus, Vitality, Shen Men, Endocrine, Adrenal Gland 1 and 2, Apex. According to TCM: Liver.

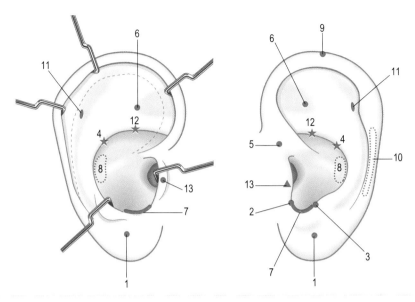

Figure 12.12 Point bank for eye symptoms.

1. Eye
2. Eye 1
3. Eye 2
4. Thymus
5. Vitality
6. Shen Men
7. Endocrine
8. Liver
9. Apex
10. Skin Disorder
11. Urticaria Groove
12. Adrenal Gland 1
13. Adrenal Gland 2

Inflammation of the eyelid

Eye (all three eye points can be treated), Liver, Apex.

Inflammation of the eye

Eye (all three eye points can be treated), Shen Men, Liver, Skin Disorder, Adrenal Gland 1 and 2, Apex, use bleeding technique.

Symptoms of the stomach and intestinal system

Rule out serious disease and poor diet.

Point bank for symptoms of the stomach and intestines

See Figs. 12.13 and 12.14.

Use active reflex points for the body parts concerned, for example, Stomach, Duodenum, Small Intestine, Large Intestine, Rectum, Liver, Pancreas, Spleen (C) and (F), Gallbladder and Abdomen. Add Thalamus and Analgesic in cases of intensive pain, for example an attack of gallstones, and Adrenal Gland 1 and 2 and Endocrine if there is inflammation. Point Zero, Solar Plexus, Hypogastric Plexus, Hypothalamus, Thalamus, Shen Men, Sympathetic Autonomic Point, San Jiao and Brain have a regulatory effect. Frustration, Master Cerebral, Aggression, and Psychosomatic are examples of points which may be treated if there are psychological reasons for the

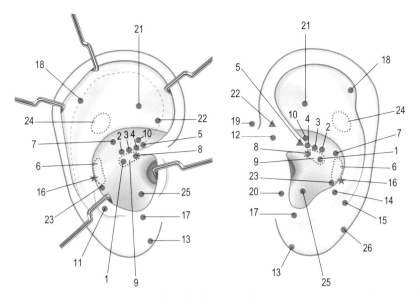

Figure 12.13 Point bank for symptoms from the stomach and intestines.

1. Stomach
2. Duodenum
3. Small Intestine
4. Large Intestine
5. Rectum
6. Liver
7. Pancreas/Spleen (F)/ Gallbladder
8. Point Zero
9. Solar Plexus
10. Hypogastric Plexus
11. Hypothalamus
12. Frustration
13. Master Cerebral
14. Neck
15. Jerome's Point
16. Muscle Relaxation
17. Aggression
18. Lesser Occipital Nerve
19. Psychosomatic
20. The V-point
21. Shen Men
22. Sympathetic Autonomic Point
23. Spleen
24. Abdomen
25. San Jiao
26. Metabolism

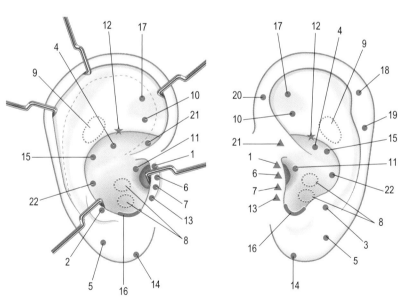

Figure 12.14 More points for symptoms from the stomach and intestines.

1. Throat (C)
2. Thalamus
3. Brain
4. Ascites
5. Inner Ear (C)
6. Inner Ear (F)
7. Master Oscillation
8. Upper and lower lung
9. Abdomen
10. Constipation
11. Throat (F)
12. Adrenal Gland 1
13. Adrenal Gland 2
14. Analgesic
15. Pancreatitis
16. Endocrine
17. Hepatitis
18. Liver Yang 1
19. Liver Yang 2
20. Haemorrhoids (C)
21. Haemorrhoids (F)
22. Cirrhosis/Hepatitis 2

symptoms. Neck, Jerome's Point, Muscle Relaxation and the V-point are examples of calming points. Specific points such as Constipation, Pancreatitis, Hepatitis, Liver Yang 1 and 2 and Haemorrhoids (C) and (F) are used if needed. Inner Ear (C) and (F) can help in cases of travel sickness.

According to TCM, the large intestine's meridian is connected to that of the lungs. For this reason the ear point Lung is used to treat intestinal symptoms. The spleen's function is, according to TCM, partly digestion of food, partly to stop leakage and 'keep things in place'. Therefore a TCM-acupuncturist will make use of the point Spleen in cases of diarrhoea, haemorrhoids and incontinence.

Bloated stomach, poor digestion

Stomach, Duodenum, Small Intestine, Large Intestine, Hypogastric Plexus, Abdomen, Point Zero, Shen Men, Sympathetic Autonomic Point, Spleen, Gallbladder, Pancreas, Solar Plexus, San Jiao, Liver, Neck, Metabolism.

Gastritis, gastric ulcer

Common reasons for this complaint are high alcohol and coffee consumption, certain medicines and smoking. Recommend a sound and well-adjusted diet, stopping smoking and a change in lifestyle if the problem is stress-related. Rule out, among other things, diaphragmatic hernia and malignancy. Consider treatment with antibiotics if there are traces of the bacteria *Helicobacter pylori*.

Point bank: Stomach, Point Zero, Shen Men, Sympathetic Autonomic Point, Hypogastric Plexus, Hypothalamus, Spleen, Duodenum, Small Intestine. Point Zero geometry: look along the lines that go from Point Zero through the reflex points for Stomach and Duodenum, in particular in the zone for the sympathetic trunk and the vegetative groove. In cases of stress and psychological complications: Frustration, Master Cerebral, Neck, Jerome's Point, Muscle Relaxation, Aggression, Lesser Occipital Nerve, Psychosomatic and the V-point.

Gastroenteritis

Think about the risk for dehydration if diarrhoea and vomiting continue for a long time. Make sure that the patient is taking enough liquids. If there is a risk that a tropical disease or parasite caused the gastroenteritis, consider making contact with a clinic specialising in infection.

Point bank: Large Intestine, Small Intestine, Rectum, Hypogastric Plexus, Point Zero, Stomach, Shen Men, Sympathetic Autonomic Point, Jerome's Point, Hypothalamus.

Nausea, vomiting

Stomach, Hypogastric Plexus, Throat, Point Zero, Solar Plexus, Shen Men, Sympathetic Autonomic Point, Thalamus, Liver, Spleen, Brain, Cerebellum, Neck.

In cases of travel sickness: Add Inner Ear (C) and (F) and Master Oscillation.

Colitis, irritable bowel syndrome

Duodenum, Small Intestine, Large Intestine, Rectum, Hypogastric Plexus, Point Zero, Abdomen, Constipation, Shen Men, Sympathetic Autonomic Point, Endocrine, Lung, Spleen, Stomach, Neck, Jerome's Point.

Constipation

Constipation can arise for many reasons. Recommend a visit to the doctor if you suspect serious illness. Several medicines give rise to constipation as a side effect. Ironically, prolonged use of laxatives can also lead to chronic constipation. Inform your patient of the benefit of a sound, regular diet, of daily exercise, sufficient intake of fluids and good toilet habits, which means breaking off what you are doing and visiting the lavatory when the intestines signal that the need has arisen. Advise your patient that prunes, linseed and plantain seeds with morning cereal and fibre-rich bread can work wonders. A carafe of water on the desk at work can be a reminder of the need to drink each day the amount of fluid which the intestines need to be able to work properly. Give ear acupuncture twice a week at first, then once a week until the intestines are working properly, or use semi-permanent needles.

Point bank: Constipation, Large Intestine, Rectum, Hypogastric Plexus, Point Zero, Sympathetic Autonomic Point, Thalamus, Spleen, Abdomen, San Jiao, Stomach, Jerome's Point, Neck.

Diarrhoea

Small Intestine, Large Intestine, Rectum, Hypogastric Plexus, Point Zero, Shen Men, Sympathetic Autonomic Point, Kidney, Neck. According to TCM: Spleen.

Haemorrhoids

Haemorrhoids (C) and (F), Rectum, Large Intestine, Thalamus, Point Zero, Adrenal Gland 1 and 2, Shen Men. According to TCM: Spleen.

Faecal incontinence

Rectum, Large Intestine, Shen Men. According to TCM: Spleen.

Gallbladder trouble

Sympathetic Autonomic Point, Shen Men, Gall Bladder, Liver, Endocrine, San Jiao, Adrenal Gland 1 and 2, Point Zero. Point Zero geometry: look along a line between Point Zero and Gall Bladder, in particular in the vegetative groove.

Gallstones: Add Thalamus and Analgesic. Give powerful stimulation to alleviate pain.

Pancreatitis, inflammation of the pancreas

Pancreas, Sympathetic Autonomic Point, Shen Men, Endocrine, Pancreatitis, Point Zero.

Hepatitis and cirrhosis of the liver

Liver, Sympathetic Autonomic Point, Spleen, Hepatitis, Liver Yang 1 and 2, Gallbladder, Shen Men, Thalamus, San Jiao, Adrenal Gland 1 and 2, Ascites, Cirrhosis.

Hiccough

Point Zero, Solar Plexus, Vagus Nerve, Sympathetic Autonomic Point, Hypothalamus, San Jiao, Shen Men, Thalamus, Liver, Neck. Point Zero geometry: look along the line which goes between Point Zero and Solar Plexus/Stomach, particularly in the zone for the sympathetic trunk and the vegetative groove.

Neurological symptoms

Point bank for neurological symptoms

See Fig. 12.15.

Treat active reflex points for the affected parts of the body. Brain, Brainstem, Cerebellum, Lesser Occipital Nerve and Thalamus are examples of reflex points for parts of the central nervous system which can be active and, if so, are worth treating. But there can be other active reflex points for the nervous system and, if so, they can also be treated. Point Zero and San Jiao regulate. Master Sensorial should be used when sensory impulses are too strong. Inner Ear (C) and (F) when the balancing system is impaired, resulting in dizziness. Shen Men, Muscle Relaxation, Neck, Master Cerebral and the V-point are examples of points with a calming effect.

According to TCM, the kidneys are closely related to the nervous system. The kidney's energy governs, among other things, the functioning of the brain and mental development. For this reason the ear point Kidney (C) is used for symptoms generated by the brain.

Also according to TCM, if the element wood is unbalanced, 'inner wind' may arise. This can express itself as dizziness, involuntary jerking or cramps. For this reason the ear point Liver is used to treat such symptoms. According to TCM, the

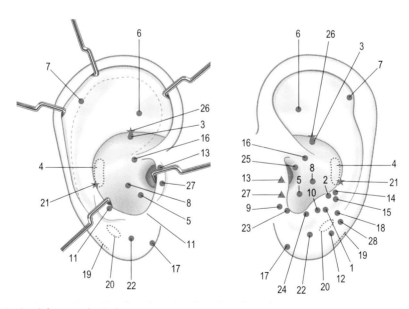

Figure 12.15 Point bank for neurological symptoms.

1. Brain	8. Heart (C)	15. Neck	22. Eye/Master Sensorial
2. Brainstem/Dizziness	9. V-point	16. Point Zero	23. Eye 1
3. Kidney	10. Forehead	17. Master Cerebral	24. Eye 2
4. Liver	11. Thalamus	18. Jaw	25. Mouth
5. San Jiao	12. Inner Ear (C)	19. Trigeminal zone	26. Adrenal Gland 1
6. Shen Men	13. Inner Ear (F)	20. Cheek	27. Adrenal Gland 2
7. Lesser Occipital Nerve	14. Cerebellum	21. Muscle Relaxation	28. Tics

heart 'opens' in the tongue, and the heart is thought to govern speech. This is why Heart (C) is used in cases of aphasia.

After a stroke

Brain, Brainstem, Kidney (C), Liver, San Jiao, Shen Men, Lesser Occipital Nerve, reflex points corresponding to the affected body parts.

In cases of aphasia: add Heart.

Dizziness

There can be many reasons for dizziness. Recommend a visit to a doctor if you suspect that the condition requires thorough medical examination. Even with such examination it can be difficult to establish the reason for dizziness and many sufferers never find out what gives rise to their condition. Take into account that dizziness can be a side effect of medication.

Point bank: Dizziness, Brain, Forehead, Shen Men, Thalamus, Lesser Occipital Nerve, Inner Ear (C) and (F), Kidney (C), Cerebellum, Neck, Point Zero, Master Sensorial, Liver.

Facial paralysis

Trigeminal Zone, Cheek, Neck, Point Zero, Shen Men, Liver, Muscle Relaxation, Eye, Eye 1 and 2, Mouth, Adrenal Gland 1 and 2, Master Cerebral, Thalamus, Brain, Lesser Occipital Nerve, the V-point.

Tics

Tics, Cheek, Eye, Eye 1 and 2, Forehead, Mouth, Jaw, Muscle Relaxation, reflex points for the cervical vertebrae, Point Zero, Shen Men, Master Cerebral, Liver.

Several neurological illnesses and symptoms are described under other headings in this chapter.

Problems with the urinary tract

Point bank for symptoms of the urinary tract

See Fig. 12.16.

Choose among active reflex points for the affected body part, for example Kidney (C) and Kidney (F), Ureter, Urinary Bladder, Urethra, Prostate and Abdomen.

Hypogastric Plexus, Thalamus, Sympathetic Autonomic Point, Point Zero, Endocrine, Hypothalamus and Brain are regulatory. Neck, Master Cerebral, Shen Men are calming. Analgesic is used when there is acute pain, like renal colic, Ovary/Testicle (C) and Ovary/Testicle (F) if a hormonal factor is involved in the symptom.

According to TCM, it is the spleen's task to keep fluids and organs in place. For this reason the ear point Spleen can be used to treat incontinence, among other conditions. One of the liver's tasks, according to TCM, is to maintain 'a free flow of qi and blood'. Thus Liver is used when 'qi and blood' stagnates and in cases of frustration. Also according to TCM, the lungs regulate water passages in the body and a sufficient level of qi in the lungs meridian is necessary so that we can let things go. This is why the ear point Lung is used when the patient cannot pass water.

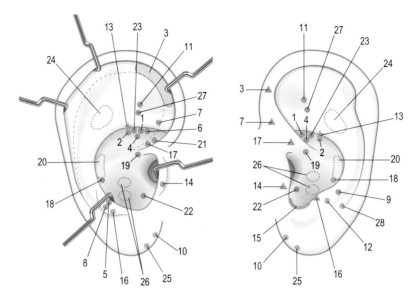

Figure 12.16 Point bank for symptoms in the urinary tract.

1. Urinary Bladder
2. Kidney (C)
3. Kidney (F)
4. Hypogastric Plexus
5. Thalamus
6. Urethra/Prostate (C)
7. Sympathetic Autonomic Point
8. Hypothalamus
9. Neck
10. Master Cerebral
11. Shen Men
12. Brain
13. Adrenal Gland (1)
14. Adrenal Gland (2)
15. Endocrine
16. Ovary/Testicle (C)
17. Ovary/Testicle (F)
18. Spleen (C)
19. Point Zero
20. Liver
21. Prostate/Vagina (F)
22. San Jiao
23. Ureter
24. Abdomen
25. Analgesic
26. Lung
27. Pelvic Girdle
28. Nephritis

Frequent urination

Urinary Bladder, Kidney (C) and (F), Urethra, Hypogastric Plexus, Thalamus, Endocrine, Point Zero, Adrenal Gland 1 and 2, Sympathetic Autonomic Point, Hypothalamus, Shen Men, Neck, Master Cerebral.

Cystitis, urinary tract infection (UTI), ureteritis

Urinary Bladder, Urethra, Kidney (C) and (F), Sympathetic Autonomic Point, Shen Men, Hypogastric Plexus, Brain, Adrenal Gland 1 and 2, Thymus.

Nephritis

Nephritis, Kidney (C) and (F), Ureter, Urinary Bladder, Sympathetic Autonomic Point, Shen Men, Point Zero, Thalamus, Brain, Adrenal Gland 1 and 2, Spleen.

Incontinence

Urinary Bladder, Kidney (C), Urethra, Ovary/Testicle (C) and (F), Brain, Thalamus, Shen Men, Sympathetic Autonomic Point, Point Zero, Hypogastric Plexus. According to TCM: Spleen.

Bedwetting, enuresis

Most children finish with nappies some time between two and four years old. Involuntary discharge of urine at night and occasionally during the day is considered normal until six or seven years of age when the child is expected to be completely 'dry'. At around 15 years of age, 1 percent of children still wet the bed. There is usually a hereditary link. Stress, anxiety and trauma can bring about or influence the symptom. In such cases psychosocial treatment can be needed. Use a mild needle technique if acupuncture needles are used. Other alternatives are: pellets, acupressure, electrical treatment with a point detector which can send a weak electrical current through the point, and laser treatment.

Point bank: Urinary Bladder, Kidney (C) and (F), Urethra, Thalamus, Shen Men, Endocrine, Point Zero, Liver, Brain, Hypogastric Plexus, San Jiao, Endocrine, Adrenal Gland 1 and 2, Hypothalamus, Neck, Sympathetic Autonomic Point.

Prostatitis

Urethra, Prostate, Ovary/Testicle (C) and (F), Shen Men, Endocrine, Point Zero, Kidney (C) and Kidney (F), Adrenal Gland 1 and 2, Urinary Bladder, Pelvic Girdle.

Kidney stones

Thalamus and Analgesic in acute cases. Kidney (C) and (F), Ureter, Urinary Bladder, Abdomen, Sympathetic Autonomic Point, Point Zero, Hypothalamus, Shen Men, Adrenal Gland 1 and 2. Point Zero geometry. Powerful stimulation over a long period (maybe a few hours) will be needed to alleviate the pain.

Urine retention

Urinary Bladder, Kidney (C) and (F), Lung, Urethra, Sympathetic Autonomic Point, Hypothalamus, San Jiao, Hypogastric Plexus.

Gynaecological functional disturbances

Point bank for gynaecological problems

See Figs. 12.17, 12.18 and 12.19.

Gynaecological functional disturbances such as painful menstruation, premenstrual syndrome (PMS) and menopausal problems can be treated with ear acupuncture. Use active reflex points for the affected body part, for example Uterus (C) and (F) Abdomen, External Genitalia (C) and (F), Breast 1 and Vagina. The most important functional point is Endocrine. Think of the Endocrine point as a larger zone containing many points which correspond to the various hormonal activities (See Chapter 8, Functional points, page 107). Look in the entire hormonal zone and treat the active points that you find there.

Other important functional points in gynaecological treatment are Ovary/Testicle (C) and (F), Breast 2, Hypothalamus, Point Zero, Sympathetic Autonomic Point, Thalamus, Vagus Nerve, Hypogastric Plexus, Brain, Shen Men, Sexual Desire, Sexual Compulsion. Prostaglandin can be used when there is pain, Adrenal Gland 1 and 2 when there is stress and inflammation.

Neck, Frustration, Aggression, Master Cerebral, Jerome's Point and the V-point are examples of relaxing points which can be used when there is psychological tension. Heart, Cardiac Plexus, Insomnia 1 and 2, Depression and Brain are used when there is a hormonal imbalance disturbing sleep and psychological wellbeing.

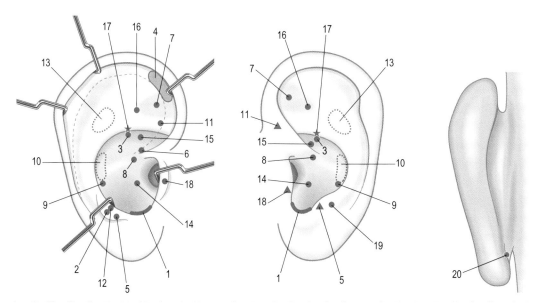

Figure 12.17 and 12.18 Point bank for gynaecological problems.

1. Endocrine
2. Hypothalamus
3. Kidney (C)
4. Kidney (F)
5. Ovary/Testicle (C)
6. Ovary/Testicle (F)
7. Uterus (C)
8. Point Zero
9. Spleen
10. Liver
11. Sympathetic Autonomic Point
12. Thalamus
13. Abdomen
14. Vagus Nerve
15. Hypogastric Plexus
16. Shen Men
17. Adrenal Gland 1
18. Adrenal Gland 2
19. Brain
20. Prostaglandin

According to TCM, the kidney's energy has great significance for fertility and reproduction. One of the liver's tasks is to provide for the free flow of qi and blood. The spleen's job is to see that fluids and organs are in the right place. Therefore the ear point Kidney (C) is used when there is disturbance in reproductive functioning, Liver when energy and blood are not circulating freely (this can show up, for example, in painful menstruation and clotting of menstrual blood, PMS, irritability and tender breasts) and Spleen when there is a large amount of bleeding, prolonged bleeding and in cases of uterine prolapse. According to TCM, the lungs manifest themselves in the skin, so if there is itching the ear point Lung should be treated.

General hormonal imbalance

Endocrine, Hypothalamus, Kidney (C) and (F), Ovary/Testicle (C) and (F).

Bleeding disturbances

Uterus, Endocrine, Shen Men, Point Zero. According to TCM: Spleen, Liver.

Painful menstruation

Uterus, Sympathetic Autonomic Point, Shen Men, Endocrine, Ovary (C) and (F), Point Zero, Hypothalamus, Thalamus (when there is acute pain), Kidney (C),

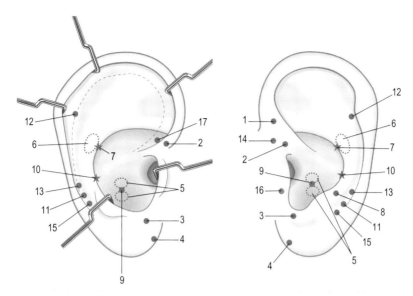

Figure 12.19 Further points used for gynaecological problems.

1. External Genitalia (C)
2. External Genitalia (F)
3. Aggression
4. Master Cerebral
5. Upper and lower lung
6. Breast 1
7. Breast 2
8. Neck
9. Heart (C)
10. Cardiac Plexus/Muscle
   Relaxation
11. Jerome's Point/Sexual
   Compulsion
12. Insomnia 1
13. Insomnia 2
14. Frustration
15. Depression
16. The V-point
17. Vagina/Prostate (F)

Abdomen, Vagus Nerve, Hypogastric Plexus, Prostaglandin, Adrenal Gland 1 and 2, Brain, Pelvic Girdle. According to TCM: Liver.

Endometriosis

Uterus, Ovary/Testicle (C) and (F), Endocrine, Shen Men, Point Zero, Adrenal Gland 1 and 2, Abdomen, Pelvic Girdle.

Amenorrhoea

See Fig. 12.19.

Uterus, Endocrine, Kidney (C), Ovary/Testicle (C) and (F), Adrenal Gland 1 and 2, Point Zero, Shen Men, Hypothalamus.

Infertility

Investigate the reasons. Stress, smoking, gross overweight, too little nourishment and too much exercise can reduce fertility. Suggest a change of lifestyle and possibly a diet supplement. If no clear reason can be found that a fertile woman has not become pregnant in a year, one can try Uterus, Ovary/Testicle (C) and (F), Point Zero, Shen Men, Hypogastric Plexus, Sympathetic Autonomic Point, Hypothalamus, Brain, active points in the Endocrine Zone, Adrenal Gland 1 and 2, External Genitalia (C) and (F). If there is psychological stress: Frustration, Aggression, Master Cerebral.

According to TCM: Kidney (C), Liver, and in cases of repeated involuntary abortions: Spleen.

Pruritus vulvae, itching of the external female genitals or the male scrotum

External Genitalia (C) and (F), Endocrine, Lung, Adrenal Gland 1 and 2, Endocrine.

Discharges

Uterus, Endocrine, Ovary. According to TCM: Kidney (C) in cases of white discharge and Liver when mixed with blood.

Tender breasts

Breast 1 and 2, Endocrine, Shen Men, Thalamus, Point Zero, Kidney, Neck.

Menopausal problems

Choose among active points those that match the most troubling symptoms.
Generally: Ovary (C) and (F), Uterus, Endocrine, Shen Men, Sympathetic Autonomic Point, Hypothalamus, Heart, Muscle Relaxation, Aggression, Frustration. According to TCM: Kidney (C), Liver.
When accompanied by perspiration: Sympathetic Autonomic Point, Hypothalamus, Lung, Brain, Adrenal Gland 1 and 2.
When accompanied by disturbed sleeping: Jerome's Point, Neck, Insomnia 1 and 2, Shen Men.
When accompanied by depression: Master Cerebral, Depression, Brain, Thalamus, Point Zero, Shen Men, Endocrine.

Premenstrual syndrome

Uterus, Ovary/Testicle (C) and (F), Endocrine, Shen Men, Point Zero, Sympathetic Autonomic Point, Hypogastric Plexus, Thalamus, Adrenal Gland 1 and 2, Brain, Kidney, Abdomen, Frustration, Aggression, Master Cerebral. According to TCM: Liver.

Impotence, frigidity, lack of libido

Sexual Desire, External Genitalia (C) and (F), Ovary/Testicle (C) and (F), Uterus, Kidney (C), Point Zero, Shen Men, Sympathetic Autonomic Point, Thalamus, Endocrine, Hypogastric Plexus, Brain, Frustration, Aggression, the V-point, Master Cerebral.

Sexually exaggerated or aggressive behaviour

Sexual Compulsion, Aggression, Ovary/Testicle (C) and (F), Thalamus, Point Zero, Shen Men.

Premature ejaculation

Sexual Compulsion, Ovary/Testicle (C) and (F), External Genitalia (C) and (F), Shen Men, Point Zero, Endocrine, Kidney (C).

Pregnancy, childbirth and breastfeeding

Take extra care in giving acupuncture to pregnant women. Most authors warn against use of the points Uterus, Ovary and Endocrine in such cases. According to others, such as gynaecologist Schulte-Uebbing (2001), there are no forbidden points so long as they are used correctly, though he points out that pregnant women should be given acupuncture by practised acupuncturists who have trained in obstetrics. Schulte-Uebbing recommends, for example, Uterus in cases of bleeding during all phases of pregnancy, during premature rupture of the membranes, the threat of premature birth and to induce delivery.

Point bank for the treatment of problems in pregnancy, childbirth and breastfeeding

See Figs. 12.20 and 12.21.

Choose among active reflex points for the part of the body concerned, for example Uterus, Lower Back, Pelvic Girdle, Abdomen, Urinary Bladder, External Genitalia (C) and (F), Urethra and Breast 1. Among applicable functional points are Ovary/Testicle (C) and (F), Breast 2, Endocrine, Sciatica, Point Zero, Brain, Shen Men, Sympathetic Autonomic Point, Hypogastric Plexus and Hypothalamus. Adrenal Gland 1 and 2 are used if there is stress. Thalamus and Analgesic are used when there is acute pain, for example birth pains.

Master Cerebral, Jerome's Point, Neck, Frustration, Aggression, Depression and Brain are good if there is psychological tension.

According to TCM, the kidney's energy has great importance not just for the functioning of the urinary tract but also for fertility and reproduction. The ear point Kidney (C) is therefore included in the treatment plan if there are problems

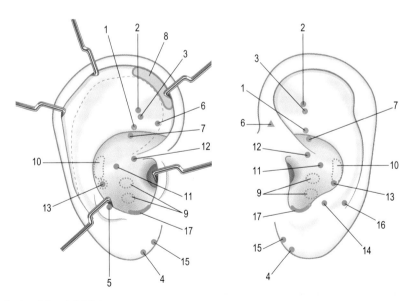

Figure 12.20 Point bank for childbirth.

1. Sciatica	6. Sympathetic Autonomic	10. Liver	15. Master Cerebral
2. Shen Men	Point	11. Stomach	16. Jerome's Point
3. Pelvic Girdle	7. Kidney (C)	12. Point Zero	17. Endocrine
4. Analgesic	8. Kidney (F)	13. Spleen	
5. Thalamus	9. Lung	14. Brain	

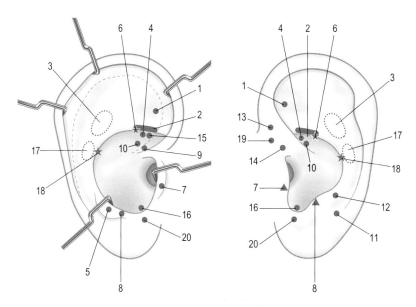

Figure 12.21 More of the points used during pregnancy, childbirth and breastfeeding.

1. Uterus (C)	6. Adrenal Gland 1	11. Depression	16. Prolactin
2. Lower Back region	7. Adrenal Gland 2	12. Neck	17. Breast 1
3. Abdomen	8. Ovary/Testicle (C)	13. External Genitalia (C)	18. Breast 2
4. Urinary Bladder	9. Ovary/Testicle (F)	14. External Genitalia (F)	19. Frustration
5. Hypothalamus	10. Hypogastric Plexus	15. Urethra	20. Aggression

with urination and certain disturbances in the reproductive function. According to TCM, the spleen makes sure that fluids and organs stay in the correct place. It is for this reason that the ear point Spleen is used to prevent uterine prolapse after birth.

Backache during pregnancy

Sciatica, Shen Men, Pelvic Girdle, reflex points for the lumbar vertebrae and for the muscles in the area. Analgesic and Thalamus in cases of acute pain.

Misuse of drugs during pregnancy

Frequent treatment with NADA, a standardised treatment that uses Sympathetic Autonomic Point, Shen Men, Kidney (C), Lung and Liver, in conjunction with supportive counselling. See Ch. 13, NADA: using ear acupuncture to fight addiction. Other points connected with craving: Craving, Master Cerebral, Jerome's Point.

Nausea during pregnancy, vomiting, morning sickness

Recommend small and frequent meals. A diet with less protein, salt and vitamin B can help. If vomiting is prolonged and there is diminished fluid intake, there can be a risk of dehydration and substantial weight loss. The mother-to-be may need an intravenous drip. Acupuncture can have a very good effect in cases of vomiting and nausea. Point bank: Stomach, Point Zero, Shen Men, Sympathetic Autonomic Point, Thalamus, Liver, Spleen, Brain, Master Cerebral, Jerome's Point.

(The body acupuncturist will add PC 6.)

Inducing childbirth

Uterus, Thalamus, reflex points for the lumbar vertebrae and for the muscles in the area, Abdomen, Point Zero, Sympathetic Autonomic Point, Shen Men, Urinary Bladder, Hypothalamus, Adrenal Gland 1 and 2, Ovary/Testicle (C) and (F), Hypogastric Plexus, Spleen. Powerful stimulation of the needles.

Delivery

Thalamus and Analgesic if there is acute pain. Tunnel from Shen Men to Uterus bilaterally with electrical stimulation or other powerful stimulation, for long periods or during successive treatments. Point Zero, Sympathetic Autonomic Point, reflex points for the lumbar vertebrae and for the muscles in the area, Sciatica, Hypogastric Plexus, Jerome's Point, Neck, Master Cerebral. Raphael Nogier suggests Omega prim, Hypothalamus and Uterus (F).

Pain after birth

Uterus, Sympathetic Autonomic Point, Shen Men, Thalamus, Analgesic, Abdomen, External Genitalia (C) and (F), Point Zero, reflex points for the lumbar vertebrae and for the muscles in the area, Spleen.

Delivery of the placenta, retained placenta

Uterus, Liver, Endocrine, Lung.

Urine retention

After childbirth it can take time for urination to function properly. Point bank: Urinary Bladder, Kidney (C) and (F), Lung, Urethra, Sympathetic Autonomic Point, Thalamus, Hypogastric Plexus, Point Zero, Neck, Jerome's Point. Stimulate every 15th minute until the bladder empties. Catheterise if the situation is acute.

Stimulating milk production

Active points in or close to Endocrine, or in the concha right above Endocrine where the point Prolactin is located, Breast 1 and 2, Shen Men. According to TCM: Spleen, Kidney.

Milk stasis, retention of milk

Empty the breast with a breast pump if necessary. (The recommendation of keeping the breasts warm is not evidence based in modern research.) Begin feeding on the painful side, and breastfeed more frequently. If improved removal of milk from the breasts does not result in improvement of symptoms over a 24-hour period, it may be advisable to seek medical opinion.

Point bank: Active points in or close to Endocrine, or in the concha directly above Endocrine where the point Prolactin is located, Breast 1 and 2. Point Zero geometry: look for active points on the line that runs between Point Zero and the Breast points, particularly in the vegetative groove. Shen Men, Sympathetic Autonomic Point, Adrenal Gland 1 and 2, Hypothalamus, Neck, Lung. If there is acute pain: Thalamus, Analgesic.

(In cases of milk retention, a body acupuncturist can also try the body points GB 41 + PC 6, or CV 17, ST 18, SI 1, GB 21.)

Postpartum depression

Recommend contact with a doctor if there are signs of serious psychological disturbance or if the mother has problems bonding with her baby. In minor cases of 'baby blues' acupuncture can help.

Try: Sympathetic Autonomic Point, Hypothalamus, Frustration, Neck, Master Cerebral, Aggression, Depression, Brain, Jerome's Point, Ovary, Endocrine.

Obesity

Several studies have shown that persons who are obese find it easier to lose weight when given ear acupuncture. Best results are achieved if the treatment is given along with dietary advice and information and encouragement to take part in physical activity. Patients should be well motivated, understand that a change in diet is necessary and willing to adopt a lifestyle that makes it possible to keep to a desired weight. Don't give rise to any unrealistic expectations. Inform patients that acupuncture is no miracle method for fast slimming. On the other hand, ear acupuncture can reduce hunger and anxiety and the desire for food, making it easier to achieve a changeover to sound and stable food habits. Encourage patients to find other ways of 'rewarding' and comforting themselves than by eating food and sweets.

Point bank for obesity

See Fig. 12.22.

Shen Men and Stomach have been used in the studies that have shown ear acupuncture to be an aid to weight loss. They reduce hunger. Other good functional points are Craving, Hunger, Hypothalamus, Hypogastric Plexus, Sympathetic Autonomic Point, San Jiao and Metabolism. Mouth can be used as a functional point to reduce oral needs. Endocrine, Pancreas and Thyroid can stabilise the hormones governing weight and appetite. Aggression, Frustration, Jerome's Point, Neck, Master Cerebral, Depression and Brain can be of use in cases of psychological tension and pent-up feelings. Nogier thought that the E-points should be given a rapid treatment (one second) before regular weight loss therapy.

According to TCM, the spleen governs the metabolism of the body, which is why the ear point Spleen is used to aid slimming. Liver is used because, according to TCM, frustrations are thought to disturb the liver's flow of qi.

Obesity

Always use the Stomach point. This reduces the feeling of hunger. Choose the most active part of the zone. Sometimes both of the points representing the upper and lower cardia are active. In such cases two needles can be inserted.

Always use Shen Men too. It calms and strengthens the psyche and enhances the effect of the other points.

Other possible points are: Craving, Hunger, Mouth, Spleen, Hypothalamus, Aggression, Hypogastric Plexus, Sympathetic Autonomic Point, Liver, Frustration, San Jiao, Endocrine, Thyroid, Pancreas, the E-points, Jerome's Point, Neck, Master Cerebral, Depression, Brain.

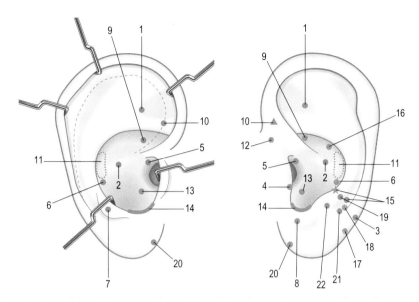

Figure 12.22 Point bank for obesity.

1. Shen Men
2. Stomach
3. Craving
4. Hunger
5. Mouth
6. Spleen (C)

7. Hypothalamus
8. Aggression
9. Hypogastric Plexus
10. Sympathetic Autonomic Point
11. Liver

12. Frustration
13. San Jiao
14. Endocrine
15. Thyroid
16. Pancreas
17. Metabolism

18. Jerome's Point
19. Neck
20. Master Cerebral
21. Depression
22. Brain

Bulimia and anorexia

Bulimia and anorexia are treated in the same way. Acupuncture is reckoned to be a balancing form of treatment which regulates the body's natural feeling of satisfaction. Use the same points as for obesity. Serious eating disturbances need psychiatric or psychosocial treatment. Acupuncture can aid treatment, not least because of its effect in dampening anxiety.

Addiction

Ear acupuncture is often included as a part of the treatment in cases of addiction on alcohol, narcotics, medicine, nicotine and other drugs (see Chapter 13, NADA: using ear acupuncture to fight addiction). Acupuncture reduces the most common withdrawal symptoms which are worry, anxiety and a craving for drugs. Most people who are given acupuncture sleep better, which gives them greater strength to get through rehabilitation. Ear acupuncture should be given as an integrated part of a treatment programme with psychosocial support. Detoxification should take place under proper supervision.

In the case of addiction to medication it can be dangerous to immediately withdraw the particular medicine. Such cases require a successive and systematic

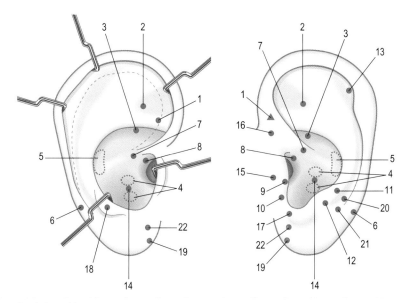

Figure 12.23 Point bank for addiction.

1. Sympathetic Autonomic Point	6. Craving	12. Brain	18. Hypothalamus
2. Shen Men	7. Point Zero	13. Lesser Occipital Nerve	19. Master Cerebral
3. Kidney (C)	8. Mouth	14. Heart (C)	20. Jerome's Point
4. Lung	9. Nicotine	15. Omega Prim	21. Depression
5. Liver	10. The V-point	16. Frustration	22. Bridging Point
	11. Neck	17. Aggression	

reduction of the dosage. At each lowering of the dosage the patient will suffer withdrawal symptoms and ear acupuncture can help the patient through these difficult periods.

During the worst of the withdrawal ear acupuncture should be given on a daily basis. Afterwards, treatment can be given at longer intervals.

Point bank for addiction

See Fig. 12.23.

Sympathetic Autonomic Point, Shen Men, Kidney (C), Lung and Liver make up the so-called NADA combination of points, most commonly used in treatment for addiction. Sympathetic Autonomic Point and Shen Men are included for their calming effect, the three other points because they represent the body's principal cleansing organs. With NADA the patient is helped through the withdrawal phase and on a good part of the long road to rehabilitation. Other possible points are Craving, Point Zero, Mouth (which in this context is used as a functional point to reduce oral need), the V-point, Neck, Jerome's Point, Brain, Lesser Occipital Nerve, the E-points (because, according to Nogier, withdrawal symptoms disturb laterality), Omega Prim (for the same reason), Frustration, Aggression, Hypothalamus, Master Cerebral, Depression, Brain, Heart and the Bridging Point.

Stopping smoking

For most smokers, quitting is a very large step to take. As with other dependencies strong motivation is decisive in achieving successful treatment. Giving information on the damage and illness to which smoking contributes is likely to have only a limited effect in getting people to kick the habit. Relapse is common. The avoidance of alcohol increases the likelihood of success in quitting smoking. For many people even coffee can generate a strong desire for a cigarette, along with sitting with other smokers. When the patient makes the sort of changes in lifestyle that are required to stop smoking, it's a good idea to suggest a form of simple exercise, walking for instance, if this is not something that he or she usually already does. Exercise reduces the risk of a relapse and counteracts a tendency to put on weight, as does a sound diet. Advise things that do not contain too much fat and sugar to put in the mouth, for example, fruit or raw carrots.

Ear acupuncture reduces the craving for nicotine. It can also create aversion symptoms: cigarettes simply don't taste the way they did before.

Common side effects when stopping smoking are strong cravings at short intervals for nicotine, disturbed sleep during the first few days, emotional instability, aggression and constipation. In the longer term, some patients become depressed and go up a few pounds in weight. Confirm that this is quite usual and explain that it will pass. Explain that nicotine gives rise to intensive but brief withdrawal symptoms as compared with many other drugs. If nicotine is not supplied in some other form (such as chewing gum, patches or tablets) the craving for it will begin to diminish after around four days. Minimise the side effects, choosing ear points liable to help what the patient considers is for the moment the worst problem. As with other such treatments for addiction, sessions should be frequent in the beginning when withdrawal symptoms are at their worst. Semi-permanent needles or pellets can be substituted between acupuncture sessions.

A good thing can be for the patient to limit smoking for a period before treatment begins. Another can be for the patient not to have smoked for several hours before the first treatment, preferably at least 24 hours. Then the patient definitely will have withdrawal symptoms and be more likely to trust the treatment as it reduces the craving.

Point bank for stopping smoking: The same as for other addictions but with the addition of Nicotine.

Psychological symptoms

Worry, anxiety, stress-related syndromes such as 'burn-out' and 'exhaustion depression', sleeping problems, depression, aggression, grief, lack of concentration and tiredness may all be treated with acupuncture to help the patient return to a stable psychological condition. Patients suffering serious psychological disturbance need psychiatric help. Ear acupuncture can be an element in such care.

Point bank for psychological symptoms

See Figs. 12.24 and 12.25.

The most common functional points in psychological treatment are Shen Men, Jerome's Point, Neck, Sympathetic Autonomic Point, Thalamus, Hypothalamus, Brain, Master Cerebral, Point Zero, Neck, Muscle Relaxation, the V-point, Aggression, Frustration and Mania. On the rear of the ear, opposite Shen Men, there

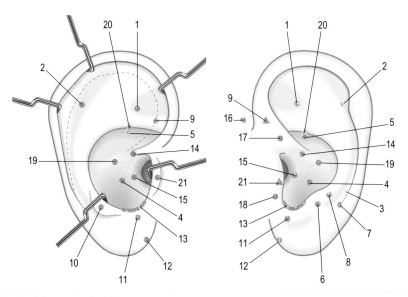

Figure 12.24 Point bank for psychological symptoms.

1. Shen Men
2. Insomnia 1
3. Insomnia 2
4. Heart (C)
5. Kidney (C)
6. Brain
7. Jerome's Point
8. Neck
9. Sympathetic Autonomic Point
10. Hypothalamus
11. Aggression
12. Master Cerebral
13. Endocrine
14. Point Zero
15. Vagus Nerve
16. Psychosomatic
17. Weather
18. The V-point
19. Stomach
20. Adrenal Gland 1
21. Adrenal Gland 2

is an excellent point which can be used to treat anxiety, preferably with pellets or seeds.

Insomnia 1 and 2 are commonly used to treat sleep disturbances. Adrenal Gland 1 and 2 can be added in cases of stress, and Depression and Brain for depression. The point Psychosomatic is thought to boost the effect of psychotherapy. Other possible additional points are Endocrine (in cases of hormonal imbalance), Weather if symptoms become worse with changes in the weather, Stomach if the anxiety seems to be located there, Vitality when the illness lasts a long time.

Nogier maintained that psychological symptoms can go together with laterality disturbance, which is why Master Oscillation can be used.

The three reflex points for the eye can be used if there are visual hallucinations as can the reflex points for the Inner Ear if the hallucinations are aural. Master Sensorial is used when sensory impulses from the surroundings become too strong.

According to TCM, depression can be caused by a disturbance in the meridians of the heart or the liver, which is why Heart and Liver are used when there is depression. According to TCM too, the kidney has a close connection with the brain's activities, which is why Kidney (C) is used if it is active.

Sleeping difficulties

First rule out the following causes of such problems: drug addiction, alcoholism, addiction to medication and serious psychological disturbance. If such is the case,

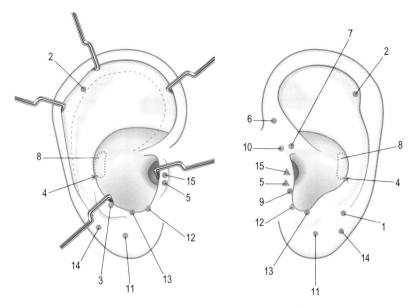

Figure 12.25 More points for treating psychological symptoms.

1. Depression
2. Lesser Occipital Nerve
3. Thalamus
4. Muscle Relaxation
5. Master Oscillation
6. External Genitalia (C)
7. External Genitalia (F)
8. Liver
9. Mania/Hunger/Nicotine
10. Vitality
11. Eye/Master Sensorial
12. Eye 1
13. Eye 2
14. Inner Eye (C)
15. Inner Eye (F)

treat the root cause. Recommend a visit to a doctor if you think this will be adequate. If the patient wakes because of a need to urinate, treat the points corresponding to the urinary tract. If the patient wakes because of pain, treat that pain. Recommend exercise and a sound diet to anyone with sleeping problems. Patients who drink a great deal of caffeine may find that they get a good night's sleep simply by changing such habits.

Point bank: Shen Men, Insomnia 1 and 2, Heart, Brain, Jerome's Point, Neck, Sympathetic Autonomic Point, Hypothalamus, Aggression, Master Cerebral, Endocrine, Point Zero, Kidney (C), Psychosomatic.

If the patient's condition worsens with a change in the weather: treat the Weather point.

Worry, anxiety

Master Cerebral, Point Zero, Shen Men, Sympathetic Autonomic Point, Brain, Heart, Jerome's Point, Neck, Hypothalamus, Psychosomatic, the V-point, Stomach, Adrenal Gland 1 and 2, Vagus Nerve.

Depression

Depression, Brain, Master Cerebral, Thalamus, Point Zero, Shen Men, Sympathetic Autonomic Point, Endocrine, Jerome's Point, Neck, Psychosomatic, Master Oscillation, External Genitalia (C) and (F). According to TCM: Liver and Heart.

Irritability

Aggression, Master Cerebral, Point Zero, Shen Men, Thalamus, Heart.

Attention deficit/hyperactivity disorder (ADHD), attention deficit disorder (ADD), deficits in attention, motor control and perception (DAMP)

Shen Men, the rear of Shen Men (by all means with pellets; see Fig. 12.26), Master Cerebral, Master Oscillation, Point Zero, Kidney (C), Brain, Neck, Jerome's Point.

Hallucinations

Shen Men, Kidney, Liver, Eye, Eye 1, Eye 2, Inner Ear (C) and (F), Brain, Master Sensorial.

'Burn-out', exhaustive depression and chronic fatigue syndrome

Shen Men, Heart, Brain, Stomach, Thalamus, Kidney, Liver, Endocrine, Vitality, Depression, Adrenal Gland 1 and 2, Point Zero, Master Cerebral, Neck, Jerome's Point.

Hysteria

Heart, Brain, Neck, Liver, Endocrine, Shen Men, Point Zero, Stomach, Kidney (C), Lesser Occipital Nerve.

Jetlag

Endocrine, Insomnia 1 and 2, Point Zero, Shen Men.

Stress

Adrenal Gland 1 and 2, the V-point, Point Zero, Shen Men, Sympathetic Autonomic Point, Master Cerebral, Muscle Relaxation, Psychosomatic, Endocrine, Neck, Jerome's Point, Liver.

Mania

Mania, Brain, Master Cerebral, the V-point, Point Zero, Shen Men, Neck, Jerome's Point, Sympathetic Autonomic Point.

Obsessive–compulsive disorder

Master Cerebral, reflex zone for the frontal lobe, the V-point, Point Zero, Shen Men, Thalamus, Heart, Neck, Jerome's Point.

Schizophrenia, psychosis

Master Cerebral, Brain, Kidney (C), Stomach, Lesser Occipital Nerve, Point Zero, Shen Men, Thalamus, Heart, Neck, Jerome's Point, Liver.

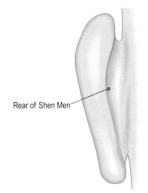

Rear of Shen Men

Figure 12.26 Rear of Shen Men.

Laterality disturbances

According to Nogier, an imbalance in the functioning of the two halves of the brain can be corrected. This means that dyslexia, depression and difficulties in concentration can be treated if they arise from such an imbalance.

Point bank and treatment suggestions for laterality dysfunction

See Fig. 12.27.

According to Nogier, ear acupuncture can be used to treat laterality disturbances using the E-points, E1 (Omega 1, Hypogastric Plexus), E2 (on the ascending helix) and E3 (near Aggression). The E-points are known as 'second points'. Begin your investigation by looking for active E-points. Look in both ears. Prick the points for one second with regular acupuncture needles if they are active. Search for active points among Omega Prim, Psychosomatic 1, Liver, Master Oscillation, Corpus Callosum, Point Zero or Shen Men and if they are active, treat them.

Nogier suggests treating Omega Prim bilaterally with a semi-permanent needle. He also suggests Liver in the right ear and Hypothalamus.

Patients with laterality problems can, according to certain theories, also benefit from other treatment. Exercises in which the patient rolls around and crawls, goes cross-country skiing or experiments with certain forms of eye movement are thought to promote collaboration between the two halves of the brain.

You can be born with laterality problems or they can arise during a period of your life. If the problem has cropped up recently, the basic reason for it must be treated and/or cleared up. A change of lifestyle may be required, a reduction of stress if that was what caused the problem, acupuncture to cure sleeping disturbances if lack of sleep caused the problem, a change or curtailing of neuroleptic drugs if it was these that caused the problem. (Curtailment of medicines should be made in consultation with the doctor who prescribed them.)

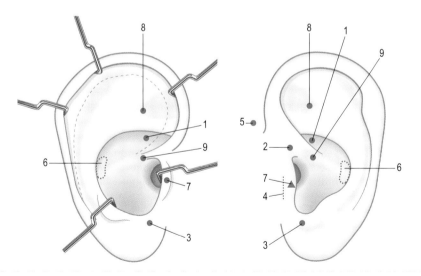

Figure 12.27 Point bank for laterality disturbances.

1. E1/Omega 1/Hypogastric Plexus
2. E2/Sexual Desire
3. E3/Pineal Gland
4. Omega Prim/Corpus Callosum
5. Psychosomatic
6. Liver
7. Master Oscillation
8. Shen Men
9. Point Zero

The point Laterality is located 3 cm in front of the ear on a level with the tragus apex and cannot be seen in the picture.

NADA – using ear acupuncture to fight addiction

The most usual procedure in ear acupuncture is to look for and treat only active points in the ear. The NADA (National Acupuncture Detoxification Association) form of ear acupuncture functions in quite another way, however. The patients are given frequent treatment using a standardised set of points (the same five points in each ear) over a long period. Initially, it was used to fight opiate addiction. Today NADA is not only used to fight many different forms of addiction, such as to alcohol, narcotics and medicaments, but also to treat worry, anxiety and sleeping difficulties. NADA is presented in a chapter of its own because this type of acupuncture is becoming more and more widespread. This standardised form of ear acupuncture is now used in more than 30 countries.

In the beginning…

The fact that acupuncture can help to reduce withdrawal symptoms was discovered quite by accident by Dr Wen, a Hong Kong neurosurgeon. Early in the 1970s he was using ear acupuncture as an anaesthetic in an operation on a patient suffering with withdrawal symptoms from opiates. He found that the acupuncture also removed the withdrawal symptoms. He repeated the experiment with several other addicts and found it worked. He wrote articles on the subject, which were read in the USA by, among others, Dr Michael Smith, a psychiatrist at the Lincoln Hospital in the South Bronx, New York. Dr Smith and his team tried and developed the method.

In the beginning, acting on the assumption that acupuncture aided withdrawal from opiates because

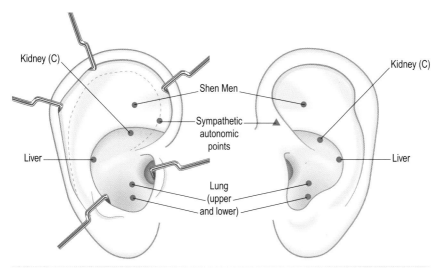

Figure 13.1 The five-points used in NADA.

it increased the release of endorphins, the body's own version of morphine, only heroin and morphine addicts were treated. The theory was that the endorphins released by acupuncture occupied the opioid receptors in the patient, thus greatly reducing withdrawal symptoms. At the Lincoln clinic staff experimented with different points in the ear and came up with the five-point combination that is today known worldwide as NADA. At each treatment session needles are inserted in five points in both ears. The points used are Sympathetic Autonomic Point, Shen Men, Kidney (C), Lung and Liver (see Fig. 13.1).

During the first year electricity was used to stimulate the needles. (Wen had done this because it was the custom when preparing a patient for an operation.) Electrical stimulation was dropped when it was found that a long-term alleviation of withdrawal symptoms could be achieved equally well without it.

The spread of NADA

Orthodox medical opinion in the 1970s was sceptical concerning the controversial ear acupuncture treatment practised by the Lincoln clinic. Very little was known about acupuncture in the USA at this time. But when the authorities tried to stop it, the patients demanded that it be continued. The NADA model spread across the USA and around 40 other countries.

NADA is an acronym for National Acupuncture Detoxification Association. It is used to describe both the method and the association that promotes it. The original association was started in the USA but now has branches in several countries. These arrange instruction and conferences, publicise the method and encourage documentation of treatment results.

NADA spread to other parts of the world in the 1980s and 1990s. In Europe there are now many NADA practitioners, for example in England, Germany, Italy, Denmark and Sweden. Several eastern European countries make use of it and its use is growing in Africa, India and Australia.

NADA is used to fight all forms of drug abuse...

When the NADA model was first developed, it was used only on patients dependent on heroin and morphine. This was in the early 1970s when endorphins, the body's own morphine, had only recently been discovered. It was known that endorphins were released during acupuncture. Thus the reasoning was that acupuncture reduced opiate withdrawal symptoms. Ear acupuncture was introduced as treatment in cases of opiate addiction or when methadone dosages were being tapered down. The focus was on reducing opiate withdrawal symptoms to levels patients could withstand so that they might continue rehabilitation without a relapse.

When a number of NADA patients reported that ear acupuncture also allowed them to get by without amphetamines, the treatment began to be used on amphetamine users, despite the fact that the medical explanation concerning the effects of endorphins no longer held true. It became apparent that ear acupuncture had a greater effect than just raising endorphin levels. In 1989 Bullock et al published a study in the British medical journal *The Lancet* in which they claimed sensationally good results using ear acupuncture to treat alcohol addiction. The article was instrumental in the wider adoption of NADA for such treatment. In the second half of the 1980s, when cocaine and crack had become a major problem, NADA was also used in the treatment of such drug users. Most published NADA research has been on clients in USA using cocaine and crack.

In some countries, such as Sweden, the next group of patients to be offered NADA treatment were those who had become addicted to prescribed drugs. Although they may have taken only the low dosages prescribed by the doctor, they found it just as hard to quit as patients who had taken much higher dosages. A reduction in dosages of analgesics (medicine to relieve pain) and in particular benzodiazepines (a group of tranquilising drugs which can be strongly addictive) takes a long time and can be very painful for the patient. Using ear acupuncture, the process of gradual reduction can be achieved more rapidly. This enables more patients to cope with withdrawal so they can slowly and safely taper down the dosage, stop taking the drug and then remain drug free.

In recent years NADA has been used to treat addiction in a wider sense of the word. It can treat compulsions to gamble, to indulge in sexual abuse or to overeat, among other things. There are no specific points in the ear for different types of addiction, but NADA's point combination seems to have a positive effect on the weakness that brings on those dependencies. It fights self-destructive thinking, inner weakness and feelings of hopelessness which precede or come with abuse.

...and in all phases of rehabilitation

The letter D in NADA stands for 'detoxification' which gives the impression that it is at this stage that the treatment should be given. NADA is very effective in treating withdrawal but is by no means just used during detoxification. On the contrary, ear acupuncture is very often the thread linking *all* phases of the rehabilitation process.

Clients can start with acupuncture treatment before becoming aware of the fact that they actually are drug abusers, and before they take part in counselling and therapy sessions. Via ear acupuncture they can be given support even during the denial phase. NADA can be given to reduce anxiety and help good sleep during the motivation phase, even before patients are ready to admit addiction. NADA can also help in establishing trust between the client and the person treating him. Patients considered to be at risk can be treated with NADA before they develop a habit.

Ear acupuncture does help during detoxification. Withdrawal symptoms are markedly relieved, increasing the chance of the patient lasting out and staying 'clean'. Then, during the long rehabilitation phase which follows, acupuncture helps to keep the patient off alcohol or drugs by relieving craving, anxiety, worry, nightmares and sleeplessness and thereby preventing a relapse. NADA is a non-confrontational treatment which allows patients to get insights into themselves and bit by bit to get through the difficult phases of rehabilitation with less pain than would otherwise be the case. Patients control their own treatment. They can 'dose' themselves with acupuncture, have as intensive or mild a programme as they choose and break off when they want to. The NADA programme creates a daily structure, providing a pleasant scheduled activity that gives calm and focus, and makes it easier for the patient to follow the rest of the rehabilitation programme. The NADA programme also provides treatment in the case of relapse, encouraging patients to return to the rehabilitation plan as soon as possible.

Stress

NADA acupuncture greatly reduces stress. The combination of points used in the NADA protocol includes Shen Men and Sympathetic Autonomic Point (for a description of these points see Ch. 7, Reflex points, and Ch. 8, Functional points), the two points most often used to treat anxiety, renowned for the peaceful effect they produce. As ear acupuncture influences the parasympathetic nervous system more than the sympathetic, it gives feelings of peace. Acupuncture influences several neurotransmitters, allowing body and soul to relax. This means NADA can also play an important part in the treatment of stress-related conditions. It also has a place as a preventative measure, before the stress felt by so many nowadays can give rise to serious symptoms. NADA is used in some workplaces and even in healthcare establishments; personnel regularly treat each other using the method.

A great part of the effect of NADA treatment is that it alleviates stress, but it would be wrong to think that this is its only effect. Patients who are dependent, for example, on heroin or alcohol, know that these drugs take away stress and grow used to taking them when they feel the need for peace and inner space. That many of them choose NADA before the drug is because ear acupuncture gives more than a temporary reduction in stress. As one patient put it, 'NADA doesn't only take away the symptom, it helps me deal with the reasons why I became a junkie'.

Post-traumatic stress syndrome (PTSS)

NADA is also used to treat post-traumatic stress syndrome (PTSS; a condition that can arise after acutely traumatic events or long-term stress). For example, after the 11th September 2001 terrorist attack on New York, a crisis centre was established at St Vincent Hospital near the World Trade Center, at which NADA treatment was given to reduce the stress levels of New Yorkers.

In the first two weeks after the catastrophe more than 1000 people were given ear acupuncture. Both relatives of victims and personnel in the emergency services were offered help in this way. Four years on, the clinic was still open two days a week, for two hours, for those who wanted help via NADA to achieve inner peace and get a clearer focus on life in order to carry on in a day-to-day reality filled with sorrow and anxiety.

For someone who has suffered trauma but is not ready to work on it verbally (or hasn't been offered or can't afford counselling or psychotherapy) NADA can help to get life back on track.

Depression

Persons who are depressed without having been traumatised can also benefit from acupuncture, which provides relief by heightening spirits. NADA can also be used to boost poor self-confidence and combat feelings of hopelessness. Even a patient with inadequate self-confidence can start treatment. In the case of exhaustion depression (burn-out), NADA may be the only treatment that badly affected patients can bear. They can sit in a group of people with needles in their ears but without feeling obliged to enter into conversation.

NADA as a treatment for other psychiatric problems

NADA can be given as a complement to many other forms of treatment for diverse categories of psychiatric disorder. For example, it is difficult to find an effective treatment for patients with double diagnosis (a person suffering both from drug abuse and a psychiatric problem). NADA can be a complement in treating such cases. It cannot cure psychosis but it can make psychotic persons calmer and enable them to get by in their day-to-day existence.

There has not been a great deal of research on acupuncture as a treatment for double diagnosis or other psychiatric illnesses (research on such patients is extremely difficult). Berman & Lundberg (2002) showed in a Swedish pilot study made on psychiatric patients in state institutions that there is a connection between ear acupuncture and better mental health. They made a comparative study between a group of patients given ear acupuncture and another group given none. The inmates who were given acupuncture had a tendency to lower levels of the stress hormone cortisol. They took less antipsychotic, anxiety depressant, calming medicine and sleeping pills. Those who were given NADA acupuncture also experienced a higher degree of autonomy, along with feelings of increased inner harmony and peace.

Other clinical experience shows that patients with double diagnosis who are given ear acupuncture become calmer, sleep better and need less medicine. In patients with a tendency to paranoia and aggression, these traits become less apparent. The whole ambience in places where patients with psychiatric problems are treated, or in forensic or custodial care, becomes less passive–aggressive and stressful when inmates are given ear acupuncture, say staff working in them.

The effect

NADA ear acupuncture has several effects. For patients who are extremely anxious, treatment is usually experienced as giving a great feeling of peace. Many fall asleep during treatment, particularly at the start of a series of sessions.

Many describe a feeling of relaxation and, at the same time, greater powers of inner concentration and consciousness. The quality of relaxation provided by NADA is not one allied to indifference but rather is focused and positive.

Those patients who are tired and indifferent can find themselves gaining vitality. They say they are being able to cope with things they had long ago ceased to bother with and that they get more things done than they had previously managed to do.

Serial NADA treatment sessions become more and more effective the further down the road the patient goes. The more treatments the patient is given, the more long-lasting the effects. In the beginning sessions need to be frequent. Later on they can be spaced out, yet still allow the patient to experience feelings of greater harmony.

When people talk of the benefits of NADA, the effects that are usually named first are that worry, anxiety and craving for drugs are all alleviated. In addition sleep is improved. If the patient is in the withdrawal phase, associated symptoms such as shaking, sweating, muscular cramps, vomiting and pain are diminished, along with irritability and nightmares.

When patients become calm and focused, they find it easier to deal with other parts of the rehabilitation programme.

More advantages of NADA

Standardisation

One advantage of NADA is that the treatment is standardised. The same five points in both ears are always treated. This means that the method is easy to learn. Most often instruction can be completed within one to two weeks. Without the need to look for active points, make a diagnosis and decide in which points needles should be inserted, treatment can be administered quickly and efficiently. For the same reason, documentation is more rapid than in other forms of treatment. Despite treatment being the same for everyone, a good percentage of patients experience it positively.

Group treatment

Another advantage of ear acupuncture, as compared with body acupuncture, is that the patient does not need to get undressed. Patients can be given treatment sitting and fully clothed, which saves time and space. It also makes it possible to offer acupuncture to patients who are so filled with anxiety they cannot lie still for examination. NADA is preferably given as a group treatment.

In body acupuncture the norm is for the patient to be undressed and to lie alone in a room during treatment. This rules out body acupuncture as a treatment for patients who feel so psychologically disturbed that they refuse to put themselves in such a vulnerable position. Patients with strong feelings of anxiety, paranoid traits or low self-esteem can find lying undressed on a couch unpleasant. This feeling is accentuated if they have to lie on their stomachs so they can't even see the acupuncturist and his 'armoury' of needles. Patients who are given ear acupuncture can move during treatment. This allows people who are so worried and filled with anxiety that they feel unable to lie still during a session to still enjoy the benefits of acupuncture. For such people ear acupuncture — sitting in a group, fully clothed — is the only viable form of acupuncture treatment. Group treatment makes NADA acupuncture attractive for many people.

Group treatment can also be more effective than individual treatment. The group dynamic can be a component in a treatment in which the patients participate in a relaxed and meditative condition.

Cost effectiveness

Acupuncture needles are cheap. And the fact that NADA treatment is best given to a group makes it still more cost effective. An ear acupuncturist can give several sessions an hour. The treatment can be given in simplified forms and ordinary premises may be used, such as living, waiting or dining rooms. No expensive or bulky benches or couches are required.

Reports from different projects show that the number of days patients with addiction or a psychiatric diagnosis need to be in hospital per year is reduced if they are given NADA as outpatients. Savings on hospital costs exceed the costs of NADA treatment.

A non-verbal treatment

NADA should be *part* of a treatment programme. Most treatment programmes for drug abuse or psychiatric problems are based on verbal therapy. NADA works without the need for talk and represents the non-verbal part of the treatment. Ear acupuncture is given freely and unconditionally, often over long periods. It can be a way to keep on board patients who, for one reason or another, find verbal therapy impossible until such time as they are ready for it. NADA gives the therapist the possibility of reaching patients who are in such poor shape or so depressed that they can't cope with talking. A patient may be afraid, unable to enter into a relationship with personnel, yet in need of treatment. Such a patient can still be given acupuncture. Many personnel value NADA precisely because it is a concrete aid that can give immediate relief from symptoms. It calms the patient and with that calm comes a realisation that relaxation is possible without chemical influence. Such a realisation may often be the reason why the patient dares to continue to take part in the rehabilitation programme.

To go straight into verbal treatment with a client who is not ready for it is scarcely very meaningful and can be a waste of resources. Ear acupuncture gives the therapist a tool he can use until such time as the patient is ready for verbal therapy. NADA prepares the way for verbal therapy and makes it more effective.

Safe, pain-free and non-addictive

Like ear acupuncture in general, NADA therapy is safe. So long as sterile needles are used in the right points in the right way, side effects are rare. People who have been or still are dependent are often used to high dosages. They lack a sensitive autonomous system. For this reason it is less likely for someone with a chemical addiction to react in a negative way to acupuncture, for example, by fainting.

On the other hand, because their receptors have been overburdened, drug addicts can be more susceptible to pain than other people. If the acupuncture is painful, it is unlikely that a patient will return. This is why NADA acupuncturists learn a light, pain-free needle technique and very few patients break off treatment because of pain.

One advantage that acupuncture has over medical treatment is that it is non-addictive, unlike many medicines used to treat withdrawal and anxiety symptoms.

Instant gratification and gradual growth

Soon after the needles are inserted in the ear, most patients feel an agreeable feeling of relaxation. Many fall asleep or into a deeply meditative condition. As a rule those who suffer most from anxiety experience the greater feelings of relaxation.

Patients feel reconciled with their thought processes and learn to let go, and have less of a tendency to brood. After a few sessions, they feel secure and draw on their own interior resources for strength and renewal. NADA improves powers of concentration and increases the ability to communicate, leaving the patient with a greater capacity to listen, learn, remember, reflect and exchange thoughts. This in turn helps to make counselling and therapy sessions, either individually or in a group, more worthwhile.

If treatment is given to a group, it creates a calming and confirming environment. It demands nothing from patients but rather allows them to work their way through their problems at their own pace.

The majority of patients feel a clear alleviation of their symptoms during NADA treatment. Others don't feel an instant gratification. Those who are patient and attend sessions on a regular basis usually experience a positive effect after a while.

Better sleep

There is a general agreement concerning ear acupuncture and sleep, with most patients reporting that they sleep better after treatment. In a rehabilitation programme this can be decisive in allowing the patient to participate fully. A good night's sleep can make fulfilment of good intentions easier to achieve.

An aid for pregnant women

NADA is a welcome aid in the treatment of addiction in pregnant women.[1] Pregnant drug users who are trying to kick their habits cannot be given tranquillisers for fear of injuring the foetus. However, NADA acupuncture can be administered safely during the entire pregnancy. Studies made in the USA and Germany show that women who have been given NADA during pregnancy have a greater likelihood of achieving a full-term pregnancy and giving birth to a baby that is not suffering from neonatal abstinence syndrome (NAS). Because women who have been given NADA give birth to healthier and sturdier babies and are more often drug-free at delivery, they will be more likely to be trusted to look after their babies themselves and to retain custody. That fewer babies are born with NAS is of great benefit for the children concerned, for their mothers and for society in general. Children born with NAS have a bad start in life, suffering withdrawal symptoms and having to be kept in an incubator, which means they are separated from their mothers. Moreover, just in terms of finance, intensive care of children with NAS, followed by their placement in foster homes (if their mothers are not drug-free and thus cannot take care of the babies themselves) costs society a great deal.

A way to cut back on on-demand medication

Clinics where NADA has been introduced report a considerable reduction in the use of on-demand medication[2] and of tranquillisers and sleeping pills in general. This is of benefit to both patients and personnel. When the patients are calmer and sleeping better, the amount of pills that have to be handed out will be greatly reduced and personnel will no longer have to deal with constant demands for extra medication.

Sometimes patients who have been given NADA ask what the needles were impregnated with before they were inserted, presuming that a chemical or drug of some kind must be involved because they have experienced such a palpable feeling of relaxation. Others say 'it feels as if I have been drinking, even though I'm

---

[1] As with other forms of acupuncture, care is recommended during pregnancy. Certain body and ear acupuncture treatment can have an influence on the uterus and should therefore not be given during the first third of the pregnancy, and sometimes not for the duration of whole pregnancy.

[2] Medicine prescribed to be given as the need arises instead of according to a fixed schedule, which can cause interminable discussions if the personnel and the patient have different opinions as to that need and a suitable dosage.

sober', or compare the acupuncture treatment with the taking of a dose of benzo-diazepine. With the realization that they have been given the same alleviation from stress that they would otherwise have experienced using drugs comes the knowl-edge that calm is to be found within. With that knowledge they can have access to the calm and sleep they need without having to ingest chemicals and the whole concept of a sober, drug-free existence becomes more meaningful, greatly boosting the rehabilitation process.

Paradoxically, several of the medicaments used in care of dependent patients are themselves addictive. Ear acupuncture provides an alternative to these, alleviating symptoms without creating new addictions. Neither does it increase tolerance levels. On the contrary, the effect of NADA treatment can be so long-lasting that the patient soon needs fewer sessions.

How treatment is given

Ear acupuncture in cases of drug addiction should be offered as a complement to other treatment. It should be given generously and without precondition to patients who want it.

It is beneficial for acupuncture to be offered to patients on a daily basis, at least during detoxification when they even may need more than one session a day. The worse the state they are in, the more important such concentrated treatment becomes. When they are in a better state ear acupuncture sessions every other day can be enough. The next stage will be twice or even once a week. After a relapse, treatment should at first be given on a daily basis again, but less frequently as the patient's condition becomes more stable.

Group treatment is thought to be more effective than individual treatment in this connection but individual treatment is better than no treatment at all.

The room

The appearance of the treatment room matters little. As to furnishing, simple chairs are all that are needed, though those with arm-rests are preferable. Models that allow the patient to lean back and relax the neck are better still.

It can be advantageous for the treatment to be given in a room where other patients can see what is happening. This usually awakens an interest in starting with the treatment themselves.

If a clinic receives NADA patients for one hour each day, at least 15 people can be treated. This may be structured as follows: when the time comes for the acupuncture session, those patients wanting treatment are let into the room. The acupuncturist begins inserting needles in the ear of the first patient while the next cleans his ears. While they wait, some of the other patients may boil water for tea and lay a tray with cups, spoons and honey.

When everyone has had needles placed in their ears and settled down in the chairs they will be sitting in for the treatment, the acupuncturist makes a round and 'fills in' any needles that might have fallen out.

Silence is golden

NADA acupuncture is a non-verbal treatment. The acupuncturist welcomes the patient and asks if everything is OK, but out of respect for the patient's integrity no more is said unless the patient starts a conversation. Of course the acupuncturist will answer questions and confirm that he or she has heard what the patient has to say.

During treatment the group is usually silent. The patients may tell one another to be quiet if someone disturbs the session, though sometimes quiet conversations may be held if the patients experience them as meaningful. They might have a great deal to learn from one another.

Music and tea

Meditative music is often used to provide a pleasant background during treatment, often in conjunction with dimmed lighting.

Patients are encouraged not to drink coffee, to smoke or to read during treatment. They are often offered herbal tea.

40-minute sessions

It is a good thing for the patients to sit with the needles in place for 40 minutes. If they want to stay longer and there is time for this, they can do so. If someone is very restless and can't sit still for such a long time, they can go earlier. When the treatment is over, the patients can remove the needles themselves or let the acupuncturist do it for them.

Motivation and connection

That the acupuncture treatment is part of a general concept is, like motivation, decisive for the final result. Each part of the programme emphasises the autonomy of the patient. Treatment is voluntary and depends upon self-responsibility for its results. The aim is 'street sobriety', the ability to keep oneself drug-free in an environment where there are drugs.

The treatment programme consists of several parts. Ear acupuncture can be the first step but may often follow the patient through the whole rehabilitation process. Other elements include support and counselling. The aim is to encourage freedom from drugs, to teach patients to deal with relapses and function socially and to get them to participate in therapy and become part of a support group.

Participation in a self-help group or network such as Alcoholics Anonymous or Narcotics Anonymous is seen as worthwhile. Contact with the group can continue for many years after a patient has been freed from addiction.

Long treatment periods

Normally, it takes around three to six months to work through the programme. During the first phase ear acupuncture relieves acute withdrawal symptoms, gives the patient peace and improved sleep. At the same time, group pressure contributes to heighten motivation should it falter. Patients say they feel calmer and have more vitality, that they think clearly and experience less anxiety and stress. Those who are given acupuncture have a greater possibility of coping with a long programme of treatment. Among those who relapse, many will seek help again at a NADA clinic.

Ear acupuncture is no miracle cure in cases of addiction but it can be a great help on the way to a sober and drug-free life.

References

Berman, A., Lundberg, U. (2002) Auricular acupuncture in prison psychiatric units: a pilot study. Acta Psychiatrica Scandinavica 106(Suppl. 412):152–157.

Bridges, L. (2004) Face reading in Chinese medicine. Churchill Livingstone, Edinburgh.

Bullock, M., Culliton, P., Olander, R. (1989) Controlled trial of acupuncture for severe recidivist alcoholism. Lancet 1(8652):1435–1439.

Carlsson, C. (1992) Grundläggande akupunktur vid smärtbehandling (in Swedish). Studentlitteratur, Lund.

Chen, J. (1982) Anatomical atlas of Chinese acupuncture points. Shandong Science and Technology Press, China. p 237–259.

Coutté, A., Zorn, A. (1988) Introduktion til auriculomedicin (in Danish). Azac forlag, Denmark.

Coutté A., Zorn, A. (1999) Auriculoterapi I och II, Vestlig öreakupunktur laerebog (in Danish). Azac forlag, Denmark.

Dale, R. (1991) Acupuncture meridians and the homunculus principle. Amer, J. Acupuncture 19:73–75.

Dale, R. (1991) The systems, holograms and theory of micro-acupuncture. Am J Acupuncture 27:207–242F.

Fu, W-K. (1975) The story of Chinese acupuncture and moxibustion. Foreign Languages Press, Beijing.

Hoffman, P. (2001) Skin disinfection and acupuncture. Acupuncture in Medicine 19(2):112–116.

Huang, H. L. tr (1974) Ear acupuncture, a Chinese medical report. The complete text by the Nanking army ear acupuncture team. Rodale Press, Emmaus, Pennsylvania.

Karavis, M. (1997) The neurophysiology of acupuncture, a viewpoint. Svensk Tidskrift för Medicinsk Akupunktur 3/97 and 4/97.

Liljequist, N. (1932) Ögondiagnosen. Allmänna delen jämte ögondiagnosens historia (in Swedish). Stockholm, Sweden.

Nilsson, L., Hemberger, L. (2004) A child is born. Doubleday, New York.

Nogier, P., Nogier, R. (1985) The man in the ear. Maisonneuve, Sainte Ruffine.

Norheim, A. J. (1994) Komplikasjoner ved akupunkturbehandling. Litteraturstudie for årene 1981–92 (in Norwegian). Tidskrift for Norsk Laegeforening nr 10 114:1192–1194.

Oleson, T. (1998) Auriculotherapy manual: Chinese and Western systems of ear acupuncture, 2nd edition, Health Care Alternatives, Los Angeles.

Oleson, T. (2003) Auriculotherapy manual: Chinese and Western systems of ear acupuncture, 3rd edn. Churchill Livingstone, Edinburgh.

Överbye, B. (1988) Frisk uten piller (in Norwegian). Hjemmenes Forlag.

Pennala, M., Pönttinen, P. J. (1985) Long term experiences in the treatment of obesity by implanted ear press needles in hypertensive patients, Acupuncture & Electro-Therapeutics Research 10:211–212.

Pöyhönen, R. (1996) Traditionell Kinesisk medicin, Del 1, Grundläggande teori (In Swedish). Svenska TCM-skolan, Sweden.

Rubach, A. (2001) Principles of ear acupuncture. Microsystem of the auricle. Thieme, Stuttgart, New York.

Schulte-Uebbing, C. (2001) Chapter title. In: Rubach A (ed) Principles of ear acupuncture. Thieme, Stuttgart, New York.

Schelderup, V. (1974) Alternativ medicin, läkekonst på nya vägar. W&W, Stockholm.

Silverstein, M E., Chang, I., Macon, N. tr (1975) Acupuncture and moxibustion, a handbook for the barefoot doctors of China, the official guide used in the countryside of China. Schocken Books, New York.

Strittmatter, B. (2003) Ear acupuncture, a precise pocket atlas, based on the works of Nogier/Bahr. Thieme, New York.

Wexu, M. (1985) The ear, gateway to balancing the body. Aurora Press, Santa Fe.

WHO (1990) Report of the working group on auricular acupuncture nomenclature. November 1990.

Xinnong, C, chief editor (1987) Chinese Acupuncture and Moxibustion, kapitlet Supplementary section, Ear Acupuncture Therapy. Foreign Languages Press, Beijing.

Bibliography

Bangming, L. (2002) Inspection of face and body for diagnoses of diseases. Foreign Languages Press, Beijing.

Bensoussan, A. (1991) The vital meridian, a modern exploration of acupuncture. Churchill Livingstone, Edinburgh.

Bick, E. (2000) Öreakupunktur (in Danish). Mnemo, Denmark.

Brumbaugh, A. (1994) Transformation and recovery, a guide for the design and development of acupuncture based chemical dependency treatment programs. Stillpoint Press, Santa Barbara.

Carlsson, C. (2002) Acupuncture mechanisms for clinically relevant long-term effects — reconsideration and a hypothesis. Acupuncture in Medicine 20(2–3):82–89.

Carnett, J. (2000) Microsystem acupuncture, University Press, iUniverse.com.

Frydenlund, J., Wiinblad, L. (2003) NADA-modellen, En indföring i öreakupunktur som behandling ved afhaengighed, misbrug og psykiatriske tilstande (in Danish). Akuskolens forlag, Denmark.

Graungaard, E. (1990) Orediagnose og öreakupunklur. In: Akupunkturens gåde (in Danish). Vist nok, Denmark.

Hagenmalm, M. (2000) Zonterapi med 20 nya punkter (in Swedish). ICA bokförlag.

Heyerdahl, L. (1991) Laerebok i akupunktur (in Norwegian). TANO, Norway.

Jayasuriya, A. (1987) Auriculotherapy. Clinical acupuncture. Medicina Alternativa International, pp 765–788.

Jiao, S. (1972) Head acupuncture. Shanxi Publishing House, Beijing.

Kho, L K. tr (1999) How to apply face, nose, hand & foot acupuncture. Medicine & Health Publishing, Hong Kong.

Lao, H H. (1999) Wrist-ankle acupuncture. Methods & applications, a new approach to the ancient therapeutic modality. Oriental Health Care Center, New York.

Lauborg, P. (1983) Introduktion i öreakupunktur (in Danish). Bokforlaget Sopela, Denmark.

Low, R. (1986) Akupunkturatlas. Minerva.

Maciocia, G. (2005) The foundations of Chinese medicine. Churchill Livingstone, Edinburgh

Mitchell, E. (1995) Fighting drug abuse with acupuncture, the treatment that works. Pacific View Press, Berkely.

Nogier, P. (1998) Handbook to auriculotherapy, 2nd edn. SATAS, Brussels.

Nogier, R. (2000) Auriculoterapi eller öreakupunktur trin 1 (in Danish). Ny Energi.

Överbye, B. (1985) Laerebok i akupunktur (in Norwegian). AB Arcanum, Göteborg, pp 189–209.

Veith, I. tr (1966) Yellow emperor's classic of internal medicine. University of California Press, Berkely.

Yau, P S. tr (1988) Scalp-needling therapy. Medicine & Health Publishing, Hong Kong.

General index

See also Point Index

Acne   78, 181
Acne rosacea   78, 181
Acquired immune deficiency syndrome (AIDS)   117
ACTH   45, 48
Active points   1, 14, 21–2, 58–9, 68, 69, 139–41, 144–7, 169, 170
Active points, choosing between   171–4
Active points, prioritising   170
Acupressure   146, 149, 159–60
Acupuncture needles   1, 3, 14, 19, 128–32, 149, 150
Acupuncture semi-permanent (ASP) needles   22, 131–2, 149, 150, 155–8, 165
Addiction   40, 90, 113, 114, 115–16, 203–5
Addiction, group treatment   137, 216
Addiction, NADA   211–20
Adrenaline   45, 47
Aggression   113, 114
Alcohol addiction   115, 120, 212–20
Alcohol swabs   149, 150–1
Allergic conjunctivitis   187
Allergic rhinitis   186
Allergy   88, 101, 106, 109, 121, 122, 180
Amalgam overload   84, 119
Amenorrhoea   107, 197
Anger   113
Angina pectoris   72, 98, 182
Animal experiments, irrelevance   39–40
Anorexia   94, 116, 203
Antihelix   63
Antitragus   64
Anxiety   74–6, 81, 83, 84, 86, 101, 106, 107, 109, 110, 207
Apex   63
Aphasia   193
Appetite   77, 94, 105, 114, 115–16, 118
Arrhythmias   84, 98, 183
Arthosis   101
Arthritis   109, 141
Ascites   120

Asthma   72, 80, 85, 88, 89, 90, 109, 114, 121, 185
Attention deficit disorder (ADD)   208
Attention deficit/hyperactivity disorder (ADHD)   110
Auriculomedicine   7–8
Autoimmune sickness   110
Autonomous nervous system   82

Back of ear   65, 70
Backache   104, 112, 177
Backache in pregnancy   200
Balance   79, 82, 83
Balancing effect   70, 105
Bedwetting   80, 81, 82, 109, 195
Belching   92
Bladder   110
Bleeding technique   3–4, 15–16, 134, 149, 161
Bleeding, treatment causing   166
Bloated stomach   190
Blood pressure   81, 86, 98, 101, 105, 109, 120–1, 182–3
Blood vessels   57–8
Bloodshot eyes   77
Body and ear acupuncture compared   21–6
Bradycardia   183
Brain, cross-section   79
Breastfeeding   88, 118, 198–202
Breasts, tender   198
Breathing   82, 116, 121
Bronchitis   90, 121, 185
Bulimia   116, 203
Burning the ear   7, 161

Calming   43–4, 76, 84, 110, 190
Cancer   117, 163
Case history   137, 139
Catarrh   78, 90
Childbirth   40, 104, 198–202
Childbirth, inducing   201
Children   164
Chinese points   59
Cholecystitis   120
Chronic fatigue syndrome   208
Circulation   97–9, 107, 141, 182

Cirrhosis   120, 191
Clamps, ear   162
Cold hands and feet   99, 182
Colds   185
Colic   83
Colitis   95, 190
Colour, skin   9, 45, 69, 141–2
Concentration difficulties   110, 208
Concha   65
Congenial faults   163
Conjunctivitis   187
Constipation   70, 95, 117, 120, 191
Contraindications   163–5
Coordination difficulties   82
Cortisol   43, 45
Coughing   72, 89, 90, 121, 185
Crohn's disease   94, 95
Cupping   16
Cystitis   101

Damp   107
Darwin's tubercle   62
De qi   19, 23–4, 39
Deformed ears   143
Degenerative diseases   163
Delivery   201
Dental problems   168
Dentistry   5, 25, 77, 112
Depression   81, 109, 110, 113, 114, 207, 208
Depression, NADA   215
Diabetes   163
Diagnosis   5, 17–19, 21
Diarrhoea   70, 84, 94, 95, 191
Differential diagnosis   22
Diffuse noxious inhibitory control (DNIC)   38
Digestion   84, 116, 117, 120, 188–91
Dizziness   74, 76, 79, 82, 83, 84, 123, 193
Dopamine   47
Drug abuse   40
Drug abuse during pregnancy   200, 218
Drug addiction   90, 212–20
Dyslexia   110, 208

Point index

Understanding the illustrations

The 'open' ear: Used to show the location of the various ear acupuncture points. Those points that are hidden when looking straight at the ear are sometimes shown in an 'open' ear. In such illustrations the edges of the helix, tragus and antitragus are folded back and held in place with hooks so that the subtragus, the inside of the antitragus and the inside of the edge of the helix become visible. In reality, no hooks would be used, of course.

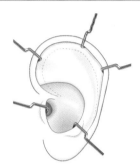

Different symbols are used to indicate the points:

● A bullet point means that the point is visible when viewed straight on.

▲ A triangle means that the point is concealed, i.e. lies on the inside of — for example — the tragus, or behind the edge of the helix.

★ A star means that the point lies on the wall between the antihelix and the concha.